The 3 M's

Motherhood, Marriage & Mental Health

Penni Fagan

The 3 M's

tellwell

Tellwell Talent
www.tellwell.ca

ISBN
978-0-2288-4490-7 (Hardcover)
978-0-2288-4489-1 (Paperback)
978-0-2288-4491-4 (eBook)

To my husband Ray, and my sons, Brayden Robert and Hank Ian. Without you three, these pages would be blank with no story to tell. Thank you for inspiring me to always get back up when I'm knocked down, for driving me completely batty, but most importantly filling my heart with endless love and laughter.

CONTENTS

Prologue ... vii

Part I. Motherhood ... 1

Anxiety's a Bitch! ... 3
Our Love Story ... 5
A Child is a Bigger Commitment than Marriage ... 8
Decision Time ... 11
Stress Isn't Good for the Baby ... 13
Home Sweet Home ... 18
It's Showtime ... 19
The Miracle of Life ... 23
Boy or Girl? ... 24
Get Me Out of Here ... 25
Why Won't My Baby Stop Crying? ... 26
Breastfeeding Is Best for Your Baby ... 28
MiLs ... 33
The Great Debate ... 36
Fitness Is Just as Good for You Mentally as It Is Physically .. 39
It Takes a Village to Raise a Child ... 40
Sex After Birth ... 42
Working-Mum Life ... 44
We Bought a House ... 47

Part II. Marriage ... 49

The Royal Engagement ... 51
Anxiety Can Be a Bastard Too ... 53
Love & Marriage ... 55

Another Baby or Long-Term Birth Control........................56
Where Did Those Nine Months Go? 57
There's No Place Like Home..59
Hypno-Birthing...61
Will This Baby Ever Come Out?...62
It's Showtime 64
Baby Number Two...67
Breast or Bottle Second Time Round?................................68
One Baby is Never Like Another..70

Part III. Mental Health..73
Life as Normal 75
I Need Help 78
Time For a Change 82
Do What You Love 83
A Change Is as Good as a Holiday 86
Work-Life Balance 91
Money Can't Buy Happiness..92
You're So Lucky Your Husband Can Babysit Your Kids 94
When Do You Know You're Done?.......................................97
The Effect Mental Health Can Have on Relationships 99
The Big O...101
The Mum's Guilt 105
Negativity Breeds Negativity...107
Control Freak...110
Self-Love 112
Triggers..114
Will I Ever Be His Priority?..118
Taking the Good With the Bad 120
My Villagers...122
The End..124

Epilogue...127

PROLOGUE

Maybe you've experienced one of the three M's in your life, or maybe none, or, like me, you've experienced all three and continue to battle with the balance of them on a daily basis. One may have led to the other, it may have been planned, it may not have been, but as I sit here and attempt to write, my boys running around me screaming at the top of their lungs, it reminds me that the combination is both physically and mentally challenging, every single day!

Now to get this straight, I am not any kind of doctor or professional mental health expert, and by no means is this a self-help book. It's just the raw and unedited take of an everyday mother dealing with what life throws at her.

Before any 'perfect-parenting police' committee members read this book and decide to judge, accusing me of not appreciating the gift that motherhood is, blah, blah, blah . . . STOP! Return this book. This is not the book for you. No way do I ever take for granted the miracle of being able to birth and care for my own children, but that doesn't mean it will all be sunshine and rainbows, even if that's what the majority of the world likes to portray on their social media pages. It's challenging, fucking exhausting, and bloody hard work, generally with no appreciation or gratitude. It is the most selfless role you'll ever play in your life, but somehow still the most rewarding. It is a time in your life when you will momentarily feel like you have lost yourself as a person, and instead have become a slave to the tiny humans you created. But those days will eventually pass, for you to come out the other side to discover and love the person you were always meant to be.

The number-one thing that motherhood has taught me is not to judge or compare myself to others, especially to snapshots that are posted on social media. It's hard, though, isn't it? While I'm sitting on the couch in my trackies ('cos they're the only thing that fit with all this extra baby weight I haven't lost, even though I've done every fad diet on the market! Go figure), a block of Top Deck in one hand (which I'll polish off in one go—shock, horror! Don't deny that you do this too), wine in the other, scrolling through multiple social media apps, wondering why I'm not more like Tanya, who is back into her pre-baby clothes a week after the birth, with her whole family in matchy-matchy outfits and her kids hugging (while I swear my boys plot to kill each other every day, or at least try their absolute hardest to piss each other off as much as possible). But I don't know what Tanya's life is really like behind that camera lens—maybe she's a raging alcoholic? Perhaps she suffers from anxiety? Perhaps the photos are all just a brave front as she hides in the pantry and cries all day? Or maybe she's just one fucking lucky bitch with a killer bod and well-behaved children! We'll always try to think of the worst-case scenario, as it will make us feel better about our own chaotic lives.

Now, don't get me wrong. I'm no queen! But it is a work in progress. After reading the books of a well-known Aussie mum about what it takes to become a true 'queen', it really did open my eyes to how much of a judgemental bitch I was. I've grown up surrounded by this type, so of course it came quite naturally to me. 'Penni, you're getting a bit podgy.' 'Penni, you're fading away to a shadow.' 'Penni, you won't amount to anything if you don't go to university.' And it goes on and on. But it wasn't until later on in life that I realised my judgements of others were only a reflection of myself. My own insecurities were leading me to think poorly of others. If anyone is different from us, we think they aren't the norm; they're weird, odd, strange, and open for judgement. We are all individuals, and our different personalities, appearances, etc. are what make us who we are. You aren't expected to gel with everyone, but just because you don't mesh with someone doesn't mean they should be the target for your judgement. And if you don't like someone for whatever reason, move on. You don't have to make a big song and dance about it. And don't even get me started on social media trolls, because that's a whole book in itself. How unhappy must someone like that be to have to bring someone else down on a public forum, hiding their own identity behind a computer screen? I'll just leave that there.

Ever since becoming a mum, I have followed numerous mummy bloggers. Some you may relate to, others you may not. Some are great to follow to find out what the latest *it* products are, others are frank and open about the challenges of motherhood and are even brave and kind enough to share their personal battles with mental illness. Since experiencing anxiety and getting to a stage where I felt medication was my only option, I thought I'd like to share my story with others. I considered dedicating a specialised social media page to share my experiences, or even begin a blog, but I felt my account was best written altogether in one book, not amongst daily posts and hashtags. And to be honest, social media is somewhere I find myself burying away and hiding in when my anxiety is at its worst, and it can even make it worse on some occasions. I needed to go with the old-school approach of a good old-fashioned book. Who doesn't love cuddling up on the couch in front of the fire, wine in one hand and book in the other? Who am I kidding, that was before we had the ability to download streaming apps onto our many devices, providing us with access to almost every movie and TV series under the sun. Am I right?

But in all seriousness, I hope this book makes it onto somebody's to-read list and can be related to or even help some people reach out for support on some of those darkest days.

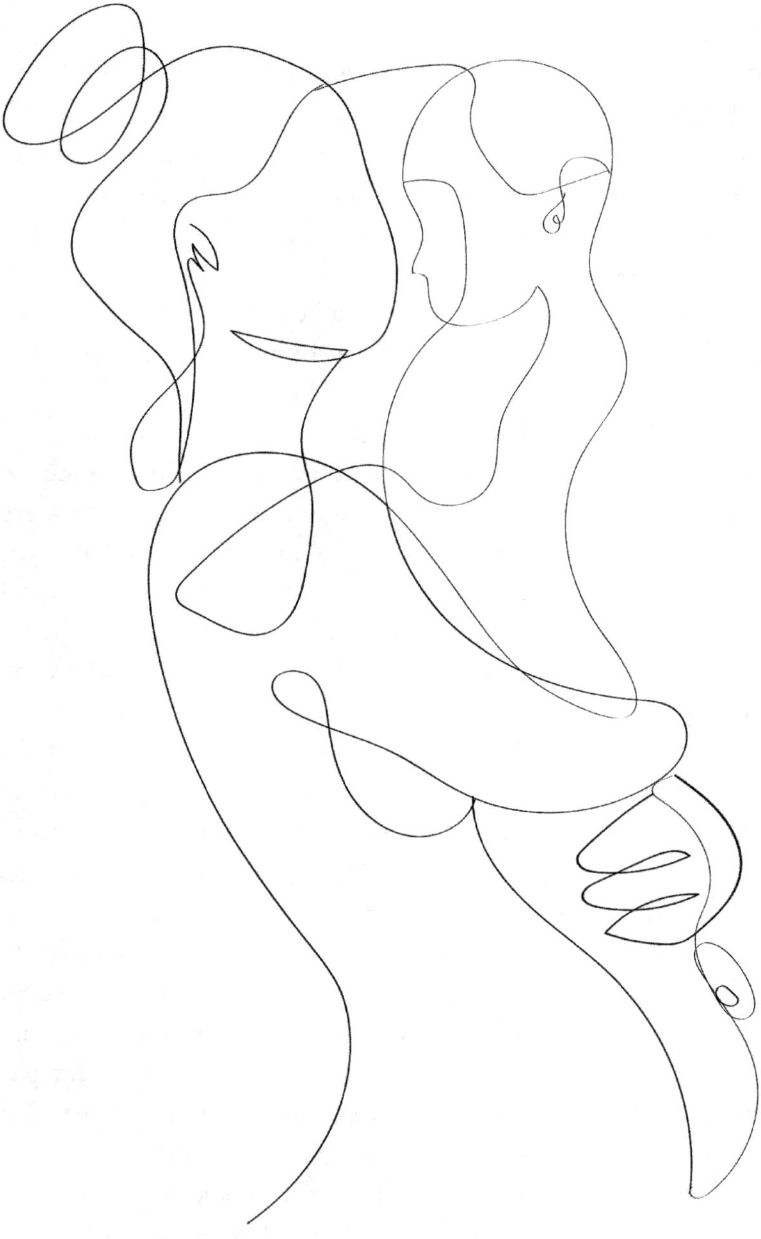

PART I

Motherhood

ANXIETY'S A BITCH!

Let's get straight to the point.

I remember one evening as if it had only happened yesterday. It was a workday for my husband; I was home with both the boys. I think my eldest was about three and my youngest six months old. I was preparing a roast for the family dinner. I had spoken to my husband earlier that day, and he had confirmed he was going to be home at a quarter to five. The kids were screaming at my feet, and I was trying to have everything perfect for when Ray arrived home. I'd been watching the clock since four p.m.! The minutes were ticking by; the kids were becoming more feral by the minute. Four forty-five came around, and I could feel it in my chest, the lump of anxiety, and right on cue my mind started racing at a hundred miles an hour. Where is he? He said he'd be home by now at the latest! The kids can feel my distress; I know they can because they want to be on me and comfort me, but I just can't deal. I message him and ask how long—no reply. He finally calls me back: 'Sorry, babe, had to drop into the boss's place and stayed for a couple beers.' I hung up and flipped out. Screaming like a wild animal that had been wounded, I picked up the roast meat and threw it against the wall, followed by the tray of vegetables, all over the kitchen walls and floor. The kids were screaming and crying; I was screaming and crying. I shut myself in the bedroom and rocked back and forth on the bed with heavy sobs. Ray arrived home to find the shit fight in the kitchen and came looking for me to ask if everything was OK. (How annoying is that question, when clearly everything isn't OK if the family dinner is painted all over the kitchen walls?) I ran out. I needed fresh air. I needed silence. I just wanted to escape what my life now was.

Even writing this paragraph, I have a feeling of tightness in my chest from reliving it. I was already seeing a counsellor, and we were already discussing and monitoring my mental state. I was always against taking medication for it and was leaving it as a last resort, trying to make life changes to reduce or overcome it naturally. I'd always been hardwired by my grandparents to just get on with it. They are from a generation that, if you are feeling down, you drag yourself out of bed and get on with your life, no excuses. Anxiety and depression were hardly spoken about in their day, but nowadays it is scarily too common. And even though I've witnessed people very close to me struggling with their own battles with mental illness, you don't quite grasp it entirely until you've lived in the dark shadows of anxiety and depression yourself.

The above incident was the last straw for me. I went straight to the doctor the following day.

People who haven't experienced anxiety before will read the above paragraph and think, *What's the big deal if he got held up for an extra half an hour? What sort of overbearing wife is she? Give the guy a break, he just wanted to have a quick beer; he deserves it after a long day's work*, and you're right. It shouldn't be a big deal, and I'm definitely not the type of wife keeping tabs on my husband's every move. But the suffocating part of anxiety is that it escalates little things like this to feel like the end of the world, seriously.

So, when did I start experiencing anxiety? How did I know my mental health was struggling? I was always so happy and outgoing to the outside world.

It wasn't until I started medication to treat my anxiety that I realised I'd probably been experiencing signs of anxiety my whole life. It just didn't get to the point that I couldn't cope with the effects of it until the joys of motherhood came my way.

OUR LOVE STORY

I didn't meet my husband until we were both in our late twenties, in the mining town of Kalgoorlie (Kal), Western Australia. We had moved to the town of pubs, skimpies and miners separately but with the same goal: to obtain jobs in the mining industry and save for the future, whatever that may be, as we both made the move alone.

We were both getting traineeships at the same mine site but at different times, and we ended up on the same crew. Ray caught my eye from the very beginning, but I could see he had caught many other girls' eyes on the same crew (he was a bit of a ladies' man!), and he was also kind of seeing someone at that time. Once that romance dwindled out, we added each other on social media and it all began from there, with a few harmless flirty messages back and forth. I made a drunken arse of myself in front of him a couple of times, and then was super shy and embarrassed about it the next day. But nothing eventuated until the annual work Christmas party.

I rocked up to the pre-party drinks at our mate's place with my eye on the prize (my husband to be . . . lol). Add some vodka to skyrocket my confidence to 'who gives a fuck', and I made my move. Now I might be being a little vague when I say 'some' vodka—I was swaying before we left pre-drinks. On our way out, Ray and I were mucking around and he shoved me, causing me to stumble onto our mates' kids' tomato plants (kill me now). Anyway, that part of the story has more relevance a little later on, so keep reading. We walked to the Christmas party, me latching on to his arm like a little lost puppy (god, I was pathetic). Arriving at the party, we saw a Christmas tree with presents under it, and I thought, *Yes, I need a photo with this tree.* Stumbling over, I decided that sitting on the presents was the way to go, and they collapsed! Nothing like making a total tool of yourself in front of all your workmates and the guy you have a crush on. (Ray led me to believe that the empty boxes I had squashed under the tree had been presents for the homeless children. He had me going for months after it, and man, did I feel bad.) Needless to say, a good friend of mine dragged my drunken arse home very early on in the night before I could get escorted out by the bouncers. Passed out cold, I somehow miraculously woke to a message from Ray at midnight asking where I was. Up I jumped, in god knows what state, and met him outside mine to walk up to the pub together.

Now, this is where the real cringe-worthy part of the story starts. Getting to the pub, surrounded by our crewmates, I—still smashed with a 'no fucks given' attitude—start pulling out my best stripper moves, using Ray as my pole. ('Somebody come get her, she's dancing like a stripper.' Who else just started singing that in their head?) Geez, I still cringe now thinking about that night, but hey, my moves must've won him over, because here we are nearly eight years later and going strong.

Now we didn't sign the deal that night. He was dragged away from stripper Penni by jealous female work friends, and I went off dancing the night away with my mates. I thought long and hard of an excuse to catch up with him again, and then, *ding-ding*, it finally came to me. The tomato plants I had squashed! Our mates made me feel super bad for crushing their kids' plants (I still to this day don't know if they were pulling my leg or were dead serious), and if Ray hadn't nudged me I would've stayed on the path, so it was only fair that he came with me to choose new plants to replace the squashed ones. I know, right? How cheesy of an idea was this, but it worked! He came and picked me up and off to Bunnings we went. He had plans after to meet mates for a few beers, so he dropped me home. I decided to head to the pub, where my dear friend and housemate at that time, Brookey Dee, was working. I told her all about him, and she convinced me to message him to come to the pub. We both had a few beers under our belt, and one thing led to another, and we found ourselves back at mine. My plan worked! (Get him drunk and took advantage—only kidding!) I still remember every bit of that night.

So that's the beginning of our love story, starting on the twelfth of December 2012. The rest is history, as they say. As we got to know each other, we realised how much we had in common. We loved old-school music, preferred the country over the city, worked as hard as we partied, and family was everything to us. We also made each other laugh—we didn't take ourselves too seriously. We gave each other shit constantly, something we still do today. I knew very early on that I was going to marry this man and he was going to be the father of my children. But that didn't mean it was all smooth sailing. Most relationships generally aren't.

A CHILD IS A BIGGER COMMITMENT THAN MARRIAGE

In the first eighteen months Ray and I were together, we spent a large portion of it apart. My goal was always to set myself up financially for the future and move on from Kal sooner rather than later. Ray's was a bit different. He had purchased a house in Kal, he had a great group of mates there, and he was making his way up at work to reach his goal of being a shovel operator. After six months of being together, I told Ray I wanted to go and work fly in, fly out (FIFO) up in the Pilbara. I was ready to move on. Ray, not in the same headspace as me, chose to stay. A couple of days into my first week away, Ray had changed his mind and he wanted to come up there too, but it was too late. The hiring boom was done and dusted (bloody men!). So we decided to stick it out for twelve months and see how we coped with the long-distance thing so I could at least get the very lucrative yearly bonus. Not that I ever let it show to Ray, but that was one of the hardest years of my life. FIFO life isn't for everyone. It's isolating, bitchy, and damn-right nasty at times. If you weren't in with the crew's clique-bitch group, then you may as well hang yourself at the gate. I don't how many times I cried myself to sleep in that year. And even though I didn't know it at the time, I think this was when my anxiety started appearing more regularly. Ray never understood.

He was in the comfort of his home, surrounded by his mates. He'd go out on weekends and I wouldn't hear from him for days after, when I'd have to make the initial contact with him. It did my head in. Was I a jealous person back then? Yes, I was! I hated myself for it, but my insecurities were through the roof, even though I was the slimmest and fittest I'd ever been. I trained every day, if not twice a day, to keep my head from going to dark places like, 'He obviously isn't calling because the girl he took home is still in bed with him.' Man, the out-there ideas my mind created in that time were unhealthy. Did I trust Ray? Well, if I was thinking things like that, I was clearly having doubts. We were still so fresh, and not having your girlfriend to come home to after a night on the piss, maybe you could be easily persuaded, craving that affection. I'll be completely honest: it wasn't until we started our family that I stopped feeling insecure. It's like I needed something else, something more important than me, more significant for him to not leave me for someone else. I alone was never going to be enough. Now I think to myself, *If he wants to lose everything we have together and have created just to fuck someone else, then he's not who I thought I married.* But I know that I'm very blessed to have found someone like Ray, even though I have to remind myself that most days.

Getting to the end of my twelve months working away, we had made the decision that if we wanted this relationship to work, I had to come back to Kal; otherwise, we were heading straight to splitsville. Luckily I had left my old pit on good terms, and they welcomed me back with open arms.

I had always been very traditional in my beliefs, and I wanted to get married before I started a family. There was a lot of history of divorce in our family, and I didn't want that for me. Since Ray and I met later on in life, I was starting to raise the whole idea of getting married, so we didn't leave it too late to start having kids. If you have ever met my husband, you would know that he is as stubborn as a mule, and even more so if it's something he feels he is getting hassled into, so I knew we weren't getting married anytime in the near future. He also had a lot of divorce in his family, and believed a child was a much bigger commitment then tying the knot. This was when we decided we'd start to try for our first child, just before I moved back to Kal full time, thinking it would take at least six months for me to fall pregnant.

Man, was I wrong! We fell pregnant first go. Now I had to return to my old job trying to hide the signs of morning sickness in prestart meetings and then break the news to my boss that I was pregnant only three months after returning. He was not impressed in the slightest, and I didn't blame him.

DECISION TIME

WA felt like it was on the other side of the world from both our families. We used our yearly leave quota up solely by going home to visit our families in Victoria and South Australia, and it wasn't cheap. I couldn't imagine having a child without my family being nearby for support. Even though Ray missed his family like crazy too, he took a little bit more convincing to agree to move back home, wherever home was going to be for us.

Our two main priorities when moving were: one, to be as close to both sides of the family as possible for visiting, and two, work availability. Now, my husband is a creature of comfort. He doesn't like change, especially if it's unpredictable. Me, I'm the opposite. I've lived overseas and moved interstate on my own without connections or a job to go to and winged it every time. It's like I thrive on the challenge. Obviously, this time was a bit different, since we would have a family to support once we moved.

The first option we threw around was to either live in Warrnambool near Ray's family and friends, or in the Riverland near my family. Either choice would put us about a seven-and-a-half-hour drive from the other side of the family. The main reason we gave this idea the flick was the lack of job opportunities in the Riverland and, well, for anyone who hasn't been to Warrnambool, its bloody freezing nearly ninety-five percent of the year. No thanks!

Onto Plan B: a town in between both states that had good work possibilities and a population of more than thirty people. This was when we stumbled across the town of Mildura, in Victoria. I briefly remember visiting the town when I was in my teens. It was the place to go for a road trip out of the Riverland. It was a larger country town with shops, nightlife, etc., so we got googling. Ray's a mad fisherman, and we had spent enough years living in the middle of the desert with a minimum of a four-hour drive to any decent water holes, so I had him sold with the sunny town of Mildura, right on the River Murray. We didn't even visit the town before we decided to move there, we just flew by the seat of our pants.

At least now we had a destination. Now to work out the nitty-gritties: a place to live and a job for Ray. It all happened to work out quite smoothly . . . I had my nan visit Mildura and view the rental properties on our behalf, and I met a businesswoman in the area whose husband owned a transport company, and they were looking for local truck drivers. Tick-tick, time to get packing!

STRESS ISN'T GOOD FOR THE BABY

I was lucky to have an uneventful start to my pregnancy. I never threw up, but I lived on packets of potato chips to ease the symptoms of morning sickness. That saltiness was the bomb! I continued operating dump trucks at work until I was about twenty weeks, and then it was getting too uncomfortable, especially the frequent toilet visits required. Work then moved me into an office position to assist the training department with paperwork.

The weeks ticked by, and we were feeling optimistic about the move. Everything was planned; we just had to wait for the time to come to implement it. Ray owned the house we lived in, so we had decided to get it ready to rent out once we moved.

At thirty weeks, I woke one morning feeling a bit off. Ray had mates around early that morning to help him fix up the backyard. I slowly dragged myself out of bed, and that's when I felt the warmness between my legs, the wetness. I quickly ran to the toilet and pulled down my underwear—it was any pregnant woman's greatest fear: blood! I proceeded to do a wee and then wiped to see brown blood on the toilet paper. My stomach dropped and my heart started to race. I ran out to get Ray's attention in the backyard. I told him I had found a bit of blood when I went to the bathroom. He tried to brush it off as something minor and said we'd go to the doctor after; he had to go back outside to help the guys. I went back and sat on the bed crying, stood back up, and there was that feeling again, the flow of liquid between my legs, but this time it was heavier, so I ran back to the bathroom. This time I needed a pad to protect my underwear—it wasn't just a few drops anymore. I tried to keep it together, but I couldn't, I was so scared. I went out and yelled at Ray through tears and told him I was going to the hospital whether he took me there or not. Our mates understood (as anyone would!), but Ray can never let other people down. I felt let down by him at that moment, and I felt his actions made me feel like I wasn't his priority. Why didn't he drop everything and carry me to the car? This was our baby's life in danger. Red means STOP . . . danger!

Ray ended up taking me, and we were rushed straight into a private room at the hospital to immediately start the examination and implement any required tests to see if I was actually in early labour or, more importantly, if the baby was in any kind of immediate danger.

I remember feeling so scared in the moment, the most frightened I'd ever felt. It was like I was a little girl again with all these big doctors around me, prodding and probing me. I was so glad Ray had changed his mind about taking me, because I don't know what I would've done without him by my side.

The tests came back, showing blood in my urine and a positive to a urinary infection. They asked me if I had noticed burning when passing urine, but I hadn't. I had felt like I was peeing more frequently over the weekend, but I thought it was all part and parcel with being heavily pregnant. Man, was I wrong! The urinary infection was the easy part to treat; the fact that it had brought on early signs of labour was the dangerous part.

After further examination, it was clear my body was experiencing contractions. I was administered a pill to stop these before I went to the next stage of labour. We were in the small country town of Kalgoorlie. If this baby was going to come today it couldn't be there, as they weren't equipped for the birth of premature babies. I would have to get airlifted to a hospital in Perth.

The doctor on call that day was an older man, and to say he made me feel uncomfortable is an understatement. He was old school and cold. The first time he proceeded to check my cervix, I felt violated. I just wanted to throw up right there and then. He spoke to me in a demeaning manner, as if I was a weak, pathetic little girl.

All I remember is that he kept yelling at me. I was getting more and more worked up, and he's yelling at me to calm down because I was making the situation worse by panicking. I tried to take a deep breath and hold it in to calm myself down. He yelled again to '*stop overreacting!*' I looked over to Ray with tears in my eyes, saying, 'I was trying to calm myself, babe, that's why I was holding my breath to slow it down.' He knew I was trying, and I could see his frustration with the doctor was the same as mine.

He kept asking if I felt pressure in my bottom area, and I did. But it's not until you actually push a baby out that you realise that pressure is like, *Holy guacamole, I think I'm giving birth out of my arsehole.* It wasn't like the slight pressure I was feeling that day. Because I said I was feeling pressure, he proceeded to roughly jam his stubby old fingers into my vagina again to check the cervix, which was one-millimetre dilated. I found out later that it can be dilated to that extent off and on without the chance of a baby coming that day.

As a precaution, I was flown to the women and children's hospital in Perth. I was freaking out even more leading up to the flight. There was no room on the plane for Ray, so I was to go alone. They gave me a sedative to calm me down before the flight and to make sure the baby would stay safe, and hopefully in the womb.

We'd been at the hospital for most of the day by this time, and this was happening around one a.m. Ray hadn't slept, and now he was going to have to make the seven-hour drive to the hospital in the middle of the night to be by my side. He amazes me how he can just drive for long distances like that without a second thought. He's stronger than me in that department. It doesn't help that I'm half bloody blind when driving at night, though, even with my glasses.

I was transported from the hospital to the airport via ambulance. A nurse did all the routine checks when I arrived. She was horrified and couldn't understand why the doctor at the hospital had proceeded to do not one but two internal examinations with the risk of making the present infection worse.

The trip was a blur as I faded in and out of consciousness, thanks to the sedative.

By the time I had arrived at the Perth hospital, the magic pill had done its thing and the contractions had stopped. What a relief! Well, that's what we thought, anyway. I had to remain on bed rest in the hospital for another forty-eight hours to monitor for any contractions reappearing.

In this time, further ultrasounds and tests were performed, and as a result the doctors found that my cervix was only eleven millimetres thick at the time. Now, I'm no doctor, so don't quote me on the particulars, but the cervix would generally still be forty millimetres at that stage of pregnancy to be able to hold the weight of the baby. So again, this put me at a high risk for having a premature baby. The doctor prescribed immediate progesterone tablets that I had to insert into my vagina twice a day, and immediate bed rest until further notice. The catch was, though: I had to remain near the hospital in Perth in case these measures weren't enough to prevent early pregnancy.

We were only weeks away from moving our whole lives interstate at this stage, and now we had doctors telling us we may not even be able to leave Perth before this baby is born. Removalists were booked, tenants were moving into our old house, and we were slowly becoming broke as fuck with all these unpredictable circumstances getting thrown our way.

So, the worst-case scenario at this stage would be that the progesterone wouldn't help to strengthen the cervix. The doctors would be concerned that the baby could come anytime in the next ten weeks, so I would have to stay in Perth and not be allowed to travel under any circumstances, especially not from one side of Australia to the other. Not only did I have to stay in Perth, but if the baby was born I would have to wait until it was of a safe age to fly interstate, all the while living somewhere in Perth, where I knew no-one! This was a terrifying scenario. Here I was, hoping to have my family by my side when the baby was born, but instead I'd be on my own in a strange city with a little cherub fighting for its life.

What made it even more challenging was that Ray had nowhere to stay near the hospital, and he felt he should go back to work until we knew more of what was going to happen to keep us financially afloat.

The best-case scenario was that I stayed on-site at the women and children's accommodation for a week with regular monitoring. If the doctors felt confident, they would grant me permission to fly to Melbourne. There I would stay with my brother and sister-in-law on strict bed rest until thirty-five weeks, so that if anything happened I was close by a hospital that could birth and care for a premature baby.

Thankfully the gods were on our side at the time, and I was granted permission to fly interstate a week later.

HOME SWEET HOME

Everything went well in Melbourne, and we were in Mildura unpacking in no time. Sitting down and doing nothing really isn't in my DNA, especially when I had a house full of boxes calling my name, and now with it safe for the baby to come any day now, my nesting began.

We started to settle in and find our way around town without needing a GPS. Well, Ray did, anyway—how that guy remembers directions after only visiting somewhere once beats me.

Moving to a new town and not knowing anyone is quite a surreal feeling. How do I meet people? How will I make friends? Work is where I had made friends in the past when moving, but this time I wouldn't be working due to a baby coming any day now.

We attended antenatal classes at the local public hospital, where we were scheduled to give birth. It was at these classes that I met my first friend in Mildura, who became a vital part of my 'village'.

The couple we met at the antenatal classes were a similar age to us. It was their first child too. Our husbands both loved fishing and a beer or two, and it was they who made the effort and offered their number for us to catch up out of the classes. I am still so grateful for that day—it made me feel like it was all going to work out.

IT'S SHOWTIME

It was a quiet Tuesday night in, I was thirty-seven weeks pregnant, the progesterone had come to an end, and baby was happy inside. Ray and I decided to have a pig out; we ordered pizza and bought a tub of ice cream.

Sprawled out on the couch in a food coma, I waddled to the toilet. When I sat to pee, I felt an odd clunk in my pelvic region. I waddled back out to the lounge room, telling Ray what had happened, slowly manoeuvring myself back onto the couch when I felt the clunk again—shit! Ray urged me to get off the couch in case I leaked on it. I jumped up, feeling warmth between my legs as a small amount of fluid ran into my underwear. Shit's starting to get real!

Had my waters just broken? In the movies, it's like floodgates opening up with litres of water gushing all over the floor; this was lucky to be fifty millilitres, if that. I thought I should call the hospital just in case. Typical Ray: 'Just sleep on it, babe. If something progresses by the morning, we'll call the hospital then.' But trusting my motherly instincts, I just knew I had to call and check in.

The nurse on the other end was calm and reassuring. It may have been my waters and it may not, so it was suggested I take my time to come into the hospital and get a check up on my progress just in case.

Generally, it can be hours or even days after your water breaks before the baby is born, but with my cervix already at a reduced thickness, I wasn't taking any chances. I went to the toilet again, and this time I felt pressure building up in my pelvic region and a dull ache in my lower back. Holy shit balls, it's happening!

The contractions came out of nowhere, and they came on strong and fast straight up, no warming up like they had led us to believe in antenatal classes. I was trying to get dressed in between sitting on the toilet, because I just had the biggest urge to shit nonstop. I had chosen the worst night ever to eat my body weight in food!

The hospital was only a ten-minute drive away, but it took an hour from that initial call to the hospital for us to arrive in between contractions, trying to get dressed and sitting on the toilet. I didn't know if I was going to even be able to make it to the hospital without shitting myself.

The car ride felt like we lived an eternity away, the contractions were strong, and sitting in a car was not making them any easier to breathe through. We pulled up to the hospital just as another contraction hit. I stood at the open car door, arms leaning on it, deep-breathing as much as I could but mainly clenching my teeth in utter pain. All I could think was, *If this is the first stage, how the fuck am I going to deal with even more pain?*

I waddled into the hospital, Ray by my side not knowing what to do, watching me bent over in pain.

We were rushed straight through the emergency department to the labour ward, where we were met by the nurse on duty. Ray explained we had called earlier; all I could do was stress that I needed a toilet, now! The urge to shit like a tap was not going away. I sat on the toilet for some relief, the nurse trying to get me to come out of the bathroom so she could check my progress, because she felt just by monitoring my pain, I was a lot further along than they would've expected. I begged to just have a quick shower before coming out for the examination. I was still shitting, standing in the shower. 'Fuck you, Penni, for eating so much just before you went into labour,' I was saying to myself. I finally got my bowels under control and lay on the hospital bed. It was so uncomfortable; all I wanted to do was sit up or bend over something. But I was new to this whole birth thing; I hadn't read all the books to know how or where you could position yourself for birth, so I lay as directed by the nurse. Now, I wasn't flat on my back—the bed was lifted at the head end—but it was still unbearable, especially once they had to put the strap around my belly to monitor the baby.

They touched on writing a birth plan in antenatal class, but I hadn't officially mapped one out. The one thing I knew was that I didn't want an epidural or caesarean unless it was the last resort to keep the baby safe. So, once I had settled and checked my cervix to see I was already four millimetres dilated, I started straight on the gas.

One of the side effects of gas, especially if you've eaten yourself stupid before going into labour, is nausea and vomiting, and that's exactly what happened. Waves of nausea swept over me, and chunky curdled pizza and ice cream came flowing out my mouth, over the side of the bed, and onto Ray's shoes. I know they say birth is the most beautiful thing, but I think they're referring mainly to holding your baby for the first time, not the stages leading up to it.

Once the initial contents of my stomach were emptied out, I continued the gas to get through the pain. I felt like I was in and out of consciousness. The waft of shit was still lingering, and I remember the nurse having to wipe away that area more than once. Real classy, Penni!

When the contractions hit I would come back to earth, lying on my side, squeezing the rails of the bed just trying to take myself anywhere but the current moment.

Ray was trying to be as nurturing as possible, but when he tried to rub my arm or touch me, I would become like the girl from the exorcist: '*Don't fucking touch me!*' so he ended up cowering in the armchair off to the side of the bed in the dark.

In one of my bouts of consciousness, I lay there and felt like everything was dark around me. I could hear echoes in the corridor, whispers of the nurses that sounded like they were miles away, but I couldn't make out what they were saying. I was staring at Ray in the chair, and the next minute a contraction hit. It was strong and it legit felt like this kid was coming out of my arsehole. I screamed at Ray, 'Where are these fucking nurses! This baby is about to come out of my arse, and they're not here!' Ray, ever so calmly while giving the nurse an apologetic smile, said, 'Babe, they're standing right behind you.' Awkward . . .

This is when the nurse did a final cervix check and finally announced it was time to push. Thank god!

Ray came to my side, keeping a bit of distance in case demon-possessed Penni resurfaced again and I started to push. During the process of pushing, the nurse asked if I wanted to hold the mirror to see the head crowning. Hell no, bitch! There is no way I wanted to see my delicate little vagina stretched to the max. I still don't know how Ray could watch his pleasure hole be ripped to shreds like that and want to jump back in after.

THE MIRACLE OF LIFE

After a short time of active labour, at one thirty a.m. our little bundle of joy was born. The baby was taken to the examination table to do the routine checks and let out a cry to let us know everything was OK. Ray carried the bundle over to the bed, all wrapped up in one of those multi-coloured hospital blankets, and laid it on my chest. I looked up at Ray and down at the amazing little human we had created. I remember looking at Ray, thinking how much more I loved him at that moment. Maybe even more than our new baby . . . is that normal? I wasn't feeling this unconditional love I had been told to expect after birth—an instant warming of my heart, bursts of uncontrollable love seeping out of me. Where were these feelings? Now, I'm not saying I didn't love my child from the beginning in that protective motherly way, but I just didn't feel *in* love.

BOY OR GIRL?

Finally, we could find out if it was a boy or a girl. We discussed at the beginning of the pregnancy if we wanted to find out the sex or not. Ray was keen to, hoping it would be a boy. I was set that I didn't want to know; I wanted that last little surprise in life kept a secret. And I didn't want Ray to know and not me, as then other people could possibly find out the sex of the baby before me. Thankfully he understood my wishes, but I always had that motherly instinct that it was a boy from the start. So much so I had even bought a navy-blue and white penguin onesie for the baby to wear when born.

And as we know, mums do know best: it was a boy. We had boy names narrowed down to two, and I was leaving it to Ray to make the final decision. He wanted to go home and sleep on it before he returned to the hospital late morning to tell me he had chosen Brayden—Brayden Robert, after Ray's dad.

The immediate family was notified. I called my nan and said, 'Would you like to come and meet your new grandson?' Silence. She couldn't believe we had only spoken the night before and he was already here. My sister even made me send her a photo, as she thought I was pulling her leg too.

GET ME OUT OF HERE

All the usual post-birth procedures were followed through with a few stitches to repair the small tear from the birth. And yes, my husband was one of those guys who made the stupid comment to the doctor, 'Can't put an extra couple of stitches in there?' Oh dear! Kill me now.

At the time of the birth, the maternity ward was being completely renovated at the hospital, meaning after the birth we were jammed into a different ward of the hospital, in a room divided into quarters, separated by curtains. Great timing! But I did choose public, not the private hospital option, so I had to deal with the situation as best I could.

After the first night of being kept awake by somebody else's baby, I had made my mind up: I was going home that day. My sister was a registered midwife and she was there to help me along the way, so I felt better cared for in the comfort of my own home.

WHY WON'T MY BABY STOP CRYING?

I feel like for the first three months of Brayden's life he cried twenty-four/seven. It may not be accurate, but at the time it felt like forever. Reliving those times now, I had anxiety then but never even thought to contemplate it as an option explaining why motherhood was so difficult for me. I was a first-time mum; of course it was meant to be hard; it's the unknown. What works for one baby might not for the next. It was so overwhelming. I used to mop my floors twice a day during that period, and straighten the towels in the guest bathroom, even though no-one was coming over. I just couldn't sit still either, all clear signs of OCD caused from anxiety.

We used to rock and shush Brayden to sleep constantly. He was never a self-settler. We tried to introduce a dummy, but initially he wouldn't take it. It wasn't until my sister-in-law let me in on one of her secret mum hacks of putting a little bit of glycerine on the end of the dummy that he took to it like a champ, which helped immensely.

I spent nights on end sleeping on the lounge with Brayden by my side or in his capsule on the floor. Having him in his bassinet in the bedroom meant endless nights without Ray getting a decent sleep and I was feeling bad, so I took camp on the couch for a week. I would watch Netflix on and off through the night between feeds and grab whatever sleep I could.

I recall during those initial months ringing Ray multiple times when he was at work in absolute hysterics because the baby just wouldn't stop crying. I'd have to put him in his cot or somewhere safe and stand outside to silence the cries just for a minute.

This next part is quite hard to write, or even admit to. It took some long contemplation on whether I wanted to leave it out of this book, but I committed to writing a raw and unedited story of a mother's life, and this is as raw as it gets. This is also the first time I've spoken out loud about it. I never hurt Brayden or was violent towards him, but during my worst times of exhaustion and frustration I did roughly place him on the change mat at times, and into his cot in the same way. I didn't throw him, but the manner in which I put him down was not acceptable by any means. I remember Ray witnessing this once or twice and wanting to say something, but he was reluctant to, knowing it would cause more tension between us, and I was already in such a mess. This is when I should've reached out for help, but I was ashamed I couldn't deal with motherhood. I was weak because I couldn't deal with my responsibilities. Why was my baby the only one that cried non-stop?

BREASTFEEDING IS BEST FOR YOUR BABY

I'd like to start this section by saying how disappointing it is to witness that, in the world today, women are still being judged by whether they breastfeed or bottle-feed their child, whether it is by nurses, doctors, other mothers, or even complete strangers. I would like to emphasise the *they*, meaning: it is *their* choice to decide what is best for their own baby. A well-fed baby is best, whether it's from a breast or a bottle. I have friends who wanted to breastfeed but couldn't due to unfortunate birth circumstances, others chose bottle from the start as it was right for them and their baby, and then I have friends who were absolute breastfeeding masters. All are amazing mums with healthy, happy children.

I gave breastfeeding my absolute best until I was forced to stop due to medical reasons. For eight weeks, I tried my hardest to try to grasp the technique and never gave up, even with a screaming baby pulling back during feeds and leaving me confused about what I was doing wrong. My husband, my nan, and my mother-in-law all tried to convince me to just switch him to the bottle. It would be easier; it would help with his feeding issues. But I was determined, because I had it drummed into my head that 'breast is best', and I had to give myself every chance to get it right.

Trying to find a solution or some sort of answer to Brayden's colic (even though doctors don't like to diagnose it as that), I made a trip to Adelaide to see a specialised osteopath with my sister. The night we arrived, I started feeling like I was coming down with a cold or something. As the next day developed, I started to feel worse from whatever I had come down with. My sister suggested I might have mastitis. I will admit I wasn't the best at checking for lumps with everything else I was dealing with at the time. I did try as much as I could to massage what I thought felt like one. I booked into a doctor the afternoon we returned home, and yes, my sister was right—I had mastitis, and it wasn't good. It had obviously gone overlooked for some time, and now I was very ill from it, and the doctor was telling me I had to go straight from the clinic to the hospital to be checked in, with an eight-week-old baby in tow.

I called Ray at work and explained the situation; he wasn't able to get off work early so I had to go straight over to emergency alone. I sat in that waiting room for hours, an anxious mum with her unsettled baby. If anyone asked me to describe hell, I think this situation would be right up there. They finally took me through into the examination cubicles, where I waited even longer. I had called my sister petrified on my way to the hospital, telling her I was on my own, and she started driving straight to Mildura. I called her again from the cubicle, wondering how far away she was, because I needed her now! She was trying to get there as quickly as possible and we both fought back the tears on the phone—hers for not being able to get there quick enough and mine for needing her to make me feel safe. She arrived and took Brayden for a walk while the doctor examined me. The doctor confirmed that yes, it was mastitis, and it had become an infected abscess that required me to be admitted to hospital straight away to begin treatment. An ongoing dose of antibiotics was needed to be injected into my body to kill off the infection before it spread any further.

Let me paint you a picture: a first-time mum with untreated anxiety now violently ill and an unsettled eight-week-old baby in a general wing of a hospital with tubes coming out everywhere. Luckily my sister was able to go home for me and grab any essentials I would need. I didn't know how long I was going to be there. I continued to breastfeed for the first couple of days in the hospital. The needle in the top of my hand that was used to transfer the antibiotics into my body was moved daily. I still didn't understand why it couldn't be in my arm, where there were more visible veins and would have made it easier for me to feed.

Unfortunately, this all happened on a Friday afternoon, so any medical assistance was limited over the weekend. A foreign-speaking surgeon did visit and unclearly spat at me that if the infection didn't go down before Monday, they would operate then. Still, they couldn't do it any earlier because it was the weekend, when they only performed emergency procedures. He also stated that if the infection had spread into my bloodstream, he would have to remove the implant in that breast too, as my body would think it was a foreign object and reject it. It was a young assistant doctor who remained in the room once the surgeon had left to translate the conversation for me to completely understand. He did reassure me that he was an excellent surgeon, even though his people skills were poor. So, to make things even worse, it was a possibility I was going to walk out with lopsided tits.

It was too late for the antibiotics to do the trick, and it was apparent early on that I was going to have the surgery performed sooner rather than later. Luckily, other patients had come into the hospital over the weekend who warranted surgery on a Sunday. It also meant Ray wasn't working either.

The surgery went off without a hitch. I was returned to my room, where a nurse was assigned to put some gauze into the wound to prevent it from closing over. The thing with an abscess in the breast when feeding is it's likely to fill back up with milk and get infected if stitched at the opening, so you have to have a huge gaping hole in your breast until the wound heals from the inside out. Unfortunately, the nurse—not knowing what she should've been doing when dressing the wound—only placed one small piece of gauze into the open hole. It was unbelievably painful, and maybe that's why she was too scared to put more in, but that's how she left it. She covered it, and it wasn't looked at again until the doctors came around the following morning to check it. They removed the bandage to see an inflamed, gaping red hole with pus in it. It was revolting. They pulled out the one piece of gauze covered in pus. This was when I realised the nurse the night before had clearly fucked up. The two doctors who cleaned out the wound that day had no mercy. I screamed so loudly during this process, and I would've had ten more babies over the pain I felt right then. They had to squirt a sterile solution into the hole to remove any infection and then pack it with an entire box of gauze, nice and tight like it should've been done initially. This was going to have to happen daily for weeks to come, until the wound slowly but surely healed from the inside out.

I was administered painkillers throughout this process, but the nurses just didn't understand how much pain I was in, or the anxiety I was experiencing. It wasn't until the second time they cleaned the wound that a female surgeon was present and could see how distressed I was. She immediately ordered them to administer more painkillers before they performed the cleaning. She was my guardian angel that day.

The first night after the operation, the anaesthetist had come in to move the needle in my hand, and he placed it in an awkward spot that restricted me from flexing my wrist up, causing pain every time I tried to pick up Brayden to feed. I pressed the assistance button to get a nurse to come. A middle-aged, overweight woman walked into the room, asking what I wanted. I was clearly already distressed and in pain, but she was making it evident from the minute she walked in the door that I was wasting her precious time. Now, I understand she was under the pump that night, understaffed and busy, but that was no excuse for the following behaviour. I explained that the needle was in an awkward position on my hand and it was painful to be able to care for my son. She went on a full rant about how she and the other nursing staff weren't there to care for my baby and how dare I even suggest such a silly thing. They had more important things to be doing. Through tears, I said I just wanted to ask if the anaesthetist could come back and move the needle. She responded by enquiring where my husband was—surely he could be caring for our child—and she stormed out. It was around two a.m. when this occurred, and I rang Ray in tears. I was pleading with him to come and take Brayden home. I got the response that he didn't know if he could get the day off work, and I shot him down by saying, 'You will come and pick your son up now; I am in hospital and not capable of caring for him. Your job will understand.'

Ray came in and took Brayden. It was then we decided to change him over to bottle feeds, since I was having so many painkillers pumped through my system it wasn't healthy for him, and hopefully it would help with the feeding issues we were having. Early that morning, the same nurse came back into my room all cheery and asked where my baby was. Can this bitch be for real? She fucking saw my husband come and grab Brayden hours ago. She looked at my wrist and, as nice as pie, stated how it was in an awkward spot; she'd get the anaesthetist to come back and reposition it. I just rolled over and didn't say a word to her.

Luckily, I wasn't in the hospital much longer after that. My wound changes were able to be performed in the comfort of my home by a visiting nurse until, evidently, I could do visits to the hospital for the last couple of weeks. Even though a scar remains to remind me of that time, the wound healed well with no long-term complications. And yes, thankfully I still have two implants in place, so no lopsided titties here.

MILS

I'd hardly spent any time with my mother-in-law before she came and stayed with Ray and me after having Brayden. Due to us living in WA for most of our relationship, visits home to see family were few and far between. We'd spoken on the phone but weren't super close due to the lack of time we'd spent together.

When my MiL came to visit, I was in the worst mental state possible. Brayden still pulled back screaming when feeding even though he had been changed to bottle feedings, and I was so self-conscious and anxious about it when anyone would visit, even family. My MiL came with only the best intentions, but I was in no way able to take on her generosity as anything but judgement.

One of the evenings my MiL stayed, I had planned on cooking a roast pork dinner. I was trying so hard to come across as the mum who had it all together in front of her, reassuring her that her son was in safe hands and well cared for. We had never cooked roast pork in the oven of our rental before, and meals we had attempted to cook told us the oven wasn't the best quality, so god knows why I decided to try to pull off pork crackling in it.

I prepared the pork and cranked up the oven to start the crackle off before lowering the temp to finish cooking the meat. Parts of the skin started to crackle and I was feeling confident it was going to work out. Once the crackle was as good as I thought it was going to get, I turned the oven down and continued to look like I had my shit together. Brayden was due to feed, so I prepared his bottle and went to sit on the lounge to feed him. To no surprise, Brayden wouldn't feed without screaming and jerking his head back. I could feel the anxiety building inside of me, even though at this time I hadn't even considered that I was struggling mentally. Brayden was feeding off my anxiousness and reflecting it in his own behaviour, and the fact that my MiL was sitting opposite me on the couch eyeballing me, wanting to take Brayden from me, made the situation a thousand times worse. I eventually had to leave the lounge room and went into the bedroom, locking the door behind me, to try to finish feeding Brayden without an audience. Our apartment wasn't big, and the sounds of Brayden's cries echoed off the walls. My MiL came knocking on the door, asking if she could take him for me. This infuriated me even more. *Why can't she just leave me alone? I left the lounge room to avoid the judgement and now she thinks she can feed my child better than I can. Who does this woman think she is?*

I yelled at her through the closed door, 'I'm fine, just leave us alone!' I eventually finished feeding Brayden and came out of the room distraught and just wanting to hide away in my room for the remainder of her stay. Ray approached me hesitantly at the stove and pleaded that his mum was just trying to help, but I just couldn't see it like that. I felt like she wanted to take over, to show me she could feed him without any issues to prove I was a useless excuse of a mother, that she knew better. Maybe deep down I was scared my son would feed without hesitation for my MiL, and I would feel rejected and even more inadequate than I already did. That the tiny bit of ego I had left would be crushed and stomped into the ground. All I needed was a break, and here she was offering me help and I just wouldn't accept it.

The crackle had gone to shit whilst I was away—something had caused the crackle that was once crispy to now be soggy. Just what I needed: not only was I incapable of feeding my own child, I couldn't cook either. I cut the skin off the roast and attempted to put it back into the oven on high heat to try to save it. No luck! I pulled it out of the oven and threw it straight into the bin. Ray came up to me and questioned why I threw it out, and I replied with a sharp, 'It's fucked.' I plated the dinner for everyone and we all sat down at the table with tension you could cut with a knife. My MiL looked around and said, 'Where's the crackle?' Ray, looking down, replied, 'Don't ask.'

At the times when we need help the most we are the least willing to accept it. No matter who it's from, sometimes it is just hard to put our egos aside and admit that, yes, their help would be amazing, even lifesaving. I should've spent that time my MiL was visiting to catch up on some much-needed sleep or enjoy the feeling of leaving the house alone, all those things I was dying to do but couldn't, since I was a first-time mum with no family living close by for daily support. The one thing I regret not doing the most during the early days of motherhood was saying yes to the help that was offered by many.

THE GREAT DEBATE

Co-sleeping: to do or not to do? This topic always stirs up controversy, especially with the risk of sudden infant death syndrome. Now, in no way do I think the risk of SIDS is to be taken light-heartedly; however, every baby is different, and with Brayden it was the difference between him waking hourly for a feed or sleeping for longer stints with the comfort of his mum. When you are sleep-deprived, you need to make the best choice for you and your baby, and Brayden was always safely placed in our bed. He didn't always sleep with us, but if he woke during the night, I'd cave and let him come in for cuddles. When I returned to work, it made things a bit harder, and we probably didn't get a solid night's sleep for at least the first eighteen months that Brayden was in our lives. I think I needed those cuddles just as much as he did, though—I loved that quiet time together where it was just the two of us, listening to his breathing, watching his beautiful little face. Brayden is five now, and I still lie with him most nights to go to sleep, or, when I'm off shift, he comes and sleeps in my bed so we can cuddle all night. And again, I think it means as much to me now, five years later, as it did in the early days of his life. I know other opinions will be quite different, because this isn't what worked for *them*, and that's OK. We all have the right to do what we feel is best for us.

Now don't get me wrong, there were times I let the opinions of others make me question my choices, second-guess myself. 'It's not safe to have your baby sleep in your bed.' 'You're only teaching him bad habits by allowing him to sleep in your bed.' 'How does your husband feel about this? It's not very fair on him.' 'Here's a book you should read on controlled crying to get your child to self-settle.' I got every judgement under the sun because I wasn't following exactly what someone else found worked for their child. And out of general fear of judgement I would try to change what worked for us, and every time it failed and broke my heart at the same time. At that time, I wasn't the mum who could just lie there and listen to my baby scream. He needed me.

I went through some really dark nights trying to change our routine. I think Brayden was about two the first time we didn't lie with him but sat by his bed and stroked his head until he went to sleep. My husband thought it was ridiculous, but it is always up to the mothers to have to change habits or routines. His thoughts made me feel guilty, and it seemed to mostly be my responsibility to do this nightly routine, so I thought it might be nice to have a child who goes to bed on his own.

The next couple of nights were torture, and the only thing that came out of it was the increased levels of anxiety I was facing. I'd put him to bed, he'd continually get back up, and I'd start getting angry and yelling, not even recognising the voice and words that were coming out of my mouth. I would sit outside the door so he couldn't get out. He would scream and scratch on the door to get out. The sounds of his screams haunt me as I write this, but at the time I felt nothing. I was numb to any emotion or reaction. This is the scary thing about mental illness: you can look back and not recognise the person you were in that moment. When you're reliving those times, it feels more like watching a movie on the big screen. Most mums will read this and think what a monster I was. And they're probably right. I've never been the perfect mother (which we should all know does not exist), but I tried my absolute best at the time. Are there times I wish I could go back and change my actions and behaviour? Every fucking day. But I can't; we can't change the past, and if we continue to live in the past our chances of becoming depressed are tenfold. All I can do is forgive myself for the mistakes I have made, learn from them and try my absolute hardest to do better in the future.

FITNESS IS JUST AS GOOD FOR YOU MENTALLY AS IT IS PHYSICALLY

I used exercise as a coping mechanism when working FIFO, and as soon as I had the all-clear from the doctor after the mastitis incident, it was my first point of call to try to start getting my shit back together. I found a small, privately owned gym that offered mum and bub sessions, and I signed up straight away. Even though I was scared shitless to walk into that class every single day, my social anxiety through the roof, I started to find some relief in the exercise, and it was the daily outing that I made sure I never missed. It was my saviour during those days, just one hour a day when I could concentrate solely on something for me, have control over something again, and lift heavy things to feel strong again, even though I was weak on the inside. I started to get some confidence back, as it didn't only help my mind, it helped me physically get back into a healthier and stronger shape.

IT TAKES A VILLAGE TO RAISE A CHILD

They say it takes a village to raise a child, and the wise person who originally said it is absolutely right! That village doesn't have to be just family; a lot of the time it is the amazing people you meet along your journey that join your village. They provide endless support and hugs; they listen without judgement and put a smile on your face when you need it the most. Without a village, motherhood can be a very lonely and scary place.

I remember getting ready for my first mums' group. I was so anxious. I wanted to look like I had my shit together, not like I lived like a slob that hardly left the house at the time because I was too petrified that Brayden would cry the whole time, and I wouldn't be able to console him in public. I even put makeup on—it's hilarious how much effort I made to hide the truth. This was where I was going to feel safe and supported, but I had already worked myself up to try to not show any cracks or weaknesses.

Walking into that room for the first time was daunting. We all looked around at each other, sussing each other out. We were a good mix of boy and girl bubs, breast- and bottle-fed, the majority around a similar age. I don't think I said much in those first few sessions; I use to be so worried about Brayden's feeding that I would heat his bottle and go into a different room to feed him, worried of the eyes and judgement that would fall on me if he started to pull back and scream, as he always still did while feeding. (Breastfeeding had nothing to do with his issues.) Everyone else's bubs were feeding away happily or sleeping.

After we got to know each other a bit better, we decided to start a group message on social media to keep in contact between sessions. It was a good way to bounce off of each other when we were having a hard time, or to organise a time to grab a coffee to hang out at the park and go for a walk to keep us all sane.

Five members of my mums' group literally saved me during that time, and all my fondest memories of the first year of Brayden's life included them. We all just got each other. We all knew we weren't perfect, but we were doing our damn bloody best to get by. We cried together; we laughed so much together that we sometimes cried again; it truly is a bond like no other. And it is where the foundation of my village really started.

Once our mothers' group sessions came to an end, we all kept in contact with weekly catchups. Everyone had that one member they were a bit closer too than the others, and mine was Ash. In the early days of adding each other on social media, we realised we had friends in common back in WA. Investigating it further, Ash had worked in human resources at the same pit I did my truck traineeship, and she had performed my initial interview. How scary is that for a small world? I'm not sure if it was having a few things in common or later living ten minutes away from each other, but Ash and I were very close friends during my time in Mildura, and we still keep in contact today. Our kids, forcibly, were best buddies too. Ash was my rock. She is your modern-day Martha Stewart with a no-bullshit approach to the world. She is the super-organised mum who always had homemade snacks on playdates and always threw the best birthday parties. She is one of the most caring and thoughtful people I know. She was there for me during thick and thin, and I am forever grateful for her non-judgemental ear and unconditional love throughout those years.

SEX AFTER BIRTH

Before I knew it, it had been six months since I had given birth and we still hadn't had sex. What made it worse was we hadn't been able to have sex for seven weeks before the birth, as advised by the doctor, due to all the potential complications. That is close to eight months of not being intimate as a couple.

I can see you all sitting there with mouths wide open, wondering how the fuck he stayed faithful to me after I hadn't put out for that long. It is a long fucking time. I know that. And it wasn't like I didn't enjoy sex before we had to stop at thirty weeks. But sometimes shit happens. Life happens.

I had a natural birth with Brayden with a few stitches that healed quite quickly, but I didn't expect the need to internally heal from birth—that would take much longer. Even though my birth was thankfully short, it was traumatic, and it wasn't until the birth of my second child that I would realise that.

It took month's post-birth for me to even be able to insert a tampon again. Everything just didn't feel right, even though medically everything had healed as expected.

The thought of trying to have sex again was always in the back of my mind, and it made me feel physically sick. I felt dirty as a person. The thought of someone touching me sexually repulsed me. When I was breastfeeding, I couldn't think of my body as anything but a mumma cow feeding her calf. My tits even hung down like cow udders when I looked at them in the mirror. My body wasn't a sexual object anymore; it was for a child to feed off and cling to for comfort. Brayden was on me constantly in those early months, and when he wasn't, I didn't want anyone or anything else to touch me. I needed to just feel the freedom of not being attached to another human being, even if it was short-lived.

Finding my sexual side again was hard. I had been at my fittest pre-birth; I was now overweight and unhealthy, in my appearance and mind. Starting back into fitness helped immensely with my self-love to try to feel like my body could belong to both a nurturing mother and a sexual woman.

It was with my mums' group that I openly spoke to about this issue, and it was their support that got me back on the horse. The first time was horrible! I felt like my insides were coming out with every single thrust. It still makes me shudder now. It took me months to try again, but with the group's hilarious way of supporting me, I got back on that horse, and this time it started to feel more normal. I still felt like my petite hole had now stretched into a wide, dark side alley, but it was a starting point.

WORKING-MUM LIFE

Once Brayden hit six months, he was instantly a better baby. It was when I started to truly fall in love with him too. Like I said before, I always loved my son in a protective motherly way, but it took time to have that undeniable adoring love for him with a bond that could never be broken. Once we were able to communicate in our own little way, through a smile, a giggle, or just cuddling having a nap on the couch, I felt the bond like no other. Finally, enjoying motherhood for all its ups and downs, I didn't have any plans to return to work so soon.

The government Centrelink parenting pay had run out, and Ray's work was on a casual basis, with hours depending on the season. We had rent to meet plus the mortgage on our house in Kalgoorlie, which we were struggling to get tenants for at the time. Ray wasn't interested in selling Kalgoorlie, nor was he keen to change jobs, and the only solution he could offer me was for him to start doing interstate driving, and at the time I just couldn't deal with him being away for nights at a time.

At this time, I felt there was no way we could keep our heads afloat without me going back to work. I had worked as a laboratory technician in wineries in my early twenties, and Mildura is surrounded by beautiful vineyards, so I thought this would be the perfect starting point. It was around October that Ray's work started slowing down, which is also when the wineries start advertising for vintage casuals to cover the harvest starting in late January and finishing up early May. I knew it wasn't full time, but it was at least a solution to get us through the next five months.

I was stoked when I received a call from a winery out in Buronga, New South Wales, only a fifteen-minute drive from where we were renting. I had put 'lab tech' as the position I was applying for, but when I arrived it was the cellar manager I met to conduct the interview with. He explained that all lab positions had been filled, but he would like to know if I was interested in a cellar-hand position. At that time, I didn't care what I was doing, as long as I was bringing money in.

I received a call a week or so later informing me that I was successful in my application and what the starting dates were. The biggest obstacle I had now was to find childcare for Brayden while working a rotating roster of days, afternoons, and nights.

Brayden was eight months old when I returned to full-time work. I was so lucky to find a lovely Indian mother who was offering family day-care and would work around my roster. For dayshifts I would drop Brayden off and pick him up, afternoons I would spend the day with Brayden and then drop him off on my way to work for Ray to pick up after his shift, and then nights Ray would drop him off on his way to work. I would pick him up once I got up just after lunch and Ray would be home before I had to leave for work. Somehow, we made it work.

Going back to work was great for my mental health too, now having adult conversations and a different role back in my life, apart from playing mum.

My first shift was at night. I hadn't slept a solid night since Brayden was born, so I was well prepared for this roster. I was introduced to an older man, and he was to be my educator and partner for the vintage, and we were inseparable by the end of it. He was like a dad figure but a mate all at the same time. We had some good laughs, and man, did it make those long nightshifts go by even quicker.

The vintage was coming to an end and casuals were getting laid off left, right and centre. They promised I was safe right up until the last few, but the cellar did not have work to keep me going until the next vintage. Knowing of my previous lab experience, the cellar manager suggested I apply for the maternity position going in the lab. He put in the best recommendation I could have ever asked for, and the job was pretty much handed to me.

After only four weeks in the lab, I was offered a full-time position. Thank god. I had a secure job locked in to cover for Ray's downtimes. The perks of changing into the lab from the cellar meant that nightshift was canned over the quiet times of the year too, so I only had to cover day and arvo shift, a win-win when it came to childcare requirements.

It was here in the lab that I met two very special villagers. One I hit it off straight away with. She had a son, just a little older than Brayden, and we just clicked from day dot. She is the most down-to-earth, funniest bitch you'll ever meet! She loves a beer or two and to get down and dirty on the dance floor. And she's there for you in a heartbeat. I am so glad our paths crossed. The second, on the other hand, was a slow-burn friendship. When I first started I felt she was a bit of a bitch to me, showing her authority, treating me like I had no idea. It's hilarious now I think back to those early days, and I can't remember what made us click, but once we did, we bonded over beers and antipasto platters at her weekly shed hangs. She is one of the most thoughtful, kind, and dear friends you could ever have. She didn't have children of her own when we met, but she just adored her friends' children. She now has a daughter who is just the cutest thing ever, and she is killing it at mum life. As I knew she always would, she's a born natural.

I think you really know who your true villagers are when they treat and love your children like they are their own.

WE BOUGHT A HOUSE

The rental we were in was way overpriced at the time, but we had no option but to accept it or we wouldn't have had a place to stay when we moved from interstate. After some time, we decided to start looking elsewhere to live. The rent we were paying could easily cover a home loan, so we reached out to a broker and found out where we sat financially to be able to buy.

We had a pre-approval done when Ray's work was busy, and I was still on Centrelink parenting payments. But when it came to us finding a lovely little weatherboard home on an acre block that we just had to have, our financers had changed. Thankfully, they were willing to take my soon-to-be employment at the winery as a safety net, and we moved into our little piece of paradise in Merbein.

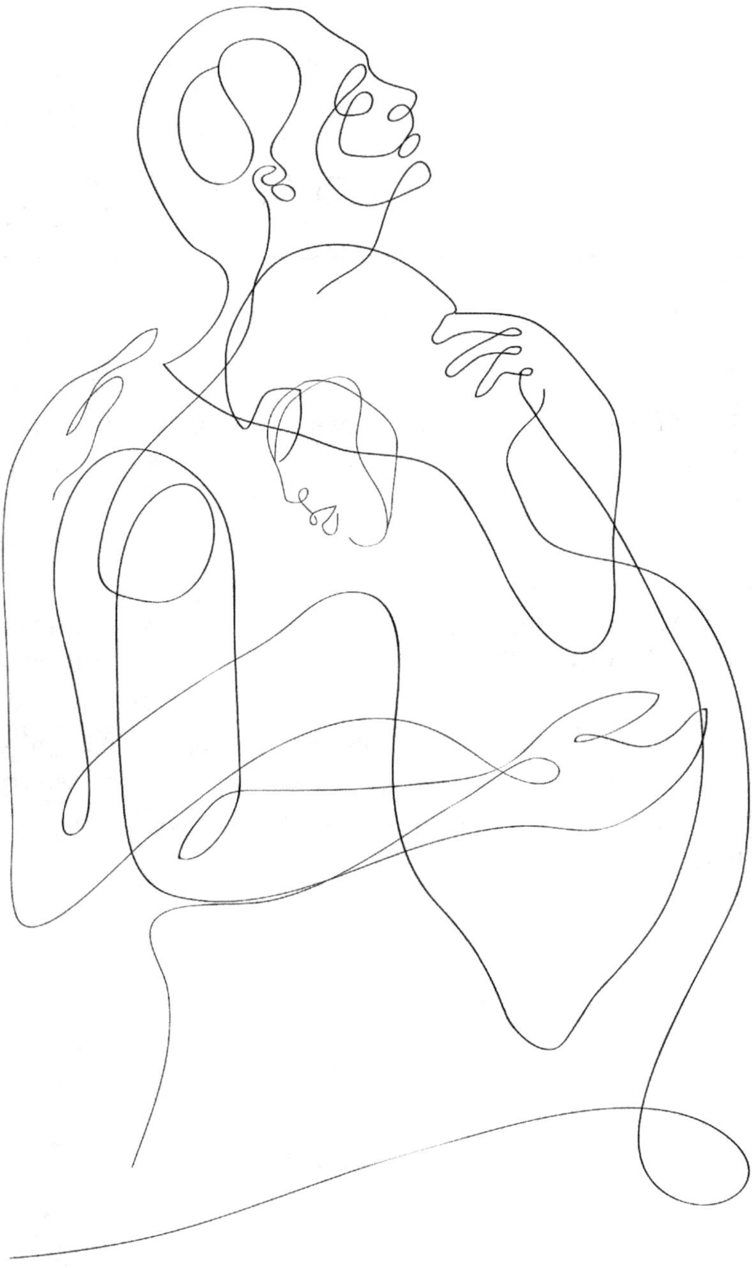

PART II

Marriage

THE ROYAL ENGAGEMENT

We bought my engagement and wedding rings long before we got engaged. When I worked for a mining company in the Pilbara, we were offered perks with local businesses for being employed by them. One was with a jeweller in Perth. I had been given a beautiful ring set from my nan from her exquisite collection when I turned thirty. She knew I wouldn't wear that particular style of ring, but proposed I use the diamonds to recreate my own. I suggested to Ray we get the rings made and take advantage of this generous discount before my employment with the company ended. If you ask Ray, he will tell you he sold his road bike for my ring—not true! But we did design the rings together, purchased the centre pear diamond, and surrounded them with my nan's diamonds. Ray put the rings in his gun safe until we moved interstate, and then he left them in the safe hands of my pop, to store in his gun safe.

In hindsight, this was the worst thing I could have done. Knowing your partner has your engagement ring and all he has to do is get down on bended knee makes you think today's going to be the day on every upcoming special occasion.

Slowly the special occasions passed by—the birth of our son, my birthday, our anniversary, Christmas, New Year's Eve—and still no proposal. Like I said earlier, if my husband ever feels he's getting pressured into doing something, he'll be even more stubborn than a mule, to prove his point that he'll do things on his terms and when he's ready. By now I'm beside myself, trying to work out why he hasn't asked me. We've got a goddamn child together for Christ's sake. Is he seriously considering not marrying me after all of this?

Easter came around, and by then I had given up hope. I was away at my grandparents for the day with Brayden, as Ray was only returning from work late that morning. He texted me to ask if I could grab the rings out of my pop's safe, as he had finally drilled his gun safe down at the new house. I didn't think any more of it and put them under the car seat to bring home. I'd been home for a bit when he asked where they were to put them in the safe, and went out to do so.

A few minutes later, a Pug-Frenchie puppy came running in the door. I had always wanted a French Bulldog, and this was the more affordable option at the time for Ray. I was like, *What the fuck is going on here?* Ray followed and lifted the puppy to me so I could see the ring around its neck. He continued to say something that I don't remember a word of, because I was lost in the moment that I had been waiting so long for. He did it on his terms, and it was a well-kept surprise. Of course I said yes.

I can see why Ray was sceptical about proposing and was holding off until he was ready, because he knew my nan and I had every little part of it planned out. We just needed the ring so we could set a date.

ANXIETY CAN BE A BASTARD TOO

Fighting my own battles with mental illness made it difficult to see the signs that Ray's mental health had also been affected by the stress of moving interstate, welcoming a child into our lives, and struggling financially. His workplace was mainly old grumpy men, and he didn't seem to form any friendships there. His carefree pre-baby freedom had come to an end, and he was restricted from going fishing and doing other things—it was hard for him to get any much-needed time on his own. I think the boat went into the water once in the first year we were in Mildura. We were both working as much as we could, with little time to play and no-one to babysit. Whenever family came to visit, we wouldn't have seen them for an extended period of time, so we felt bad asking them to look after Brayden so we could enjoy some time with just the two of us. He was starting to really dislike his job, and I just wanted him to enjoy going to work, since it was a break from the mayhem at home. I had a full-time job now, so we could afford to take the chance of Ray changing workplaces. He couldn't find anything he liked locally, and a guy at work suggested driving road trains at the sand mines up near Pooncarie. It was an hour and a half drive from us, with camp accommodation and a week-on, week-off roster. At first, I was totally against it. I had expressed to Ray when we were first together that if he wanted to do FIFO or DIDO (drive-in, drive-out) work, to do it before we had children.

He chose not to initially come with me up to the Pilbara, so for him to now decide he wanted to be away from our little family infuriated me. I eventually ended up giving in, seeing he was so unhappy. If being away from us was what he needed to change jobs and hopefully be happier, then it was something I was going to have to live with.

It was hard having him away for a week at a time, and when he would come home he was hopeless around the house. It's like it was a holiday for him to be home. Brayden would play up, and Ray would let him get away with murder, trying to make up for the week he'd just been away. This kind of lifestyle wasn't working for our family at all. It wasn't until baby number two was nearly born that I could finally convince him it was time to move home.

LOVE & MARRIAGE

Ray was right: as soon as we were engaged, Nan and I were straight onto a date for the wedding. We'd been waiting for so long to finally be able to put our plans into play, and Ray and I had already decided we wanted to get married at my grandparents' shack on the River Murray in Wigley Flat, South Australia.

Eight months after the engagement and we were married. It was one of the best days of our lives, and I wish I could relive it over and over, a hundred times again. We did have a few hurdles on the day. Our riverbank ceremony was changed to a clifftop one due to the floods that year; my arrival in a speedboat changed to me arriving in a vintage car my pop had originally built; and Brayden came down with an ear infection and was miserable the whole day, causing my grandparents to miss the ceremony as they ducked off with him in the vintage car just so we could have the perfect day. But nothing could ruin the fun. We were surrounded by our closest family and friends, beers in hand, dancing the night away with the river in the background.

As soon as the wedding was over, Ray packed his bags for his first stint, working away in Pooncarie.

ANOTHER BABY OR LONG-TERM BIRTH CONTROL

The wedding had lit a new fire between us sexually, and it was like we were in the honeymoon period all over again. I still hadn't found a pill my body was compatible with since having Brayden, and I was getting fed up trying one after the other and them all turning me loopy, especially the week leading up to my period. With periods also came unbearable cramps, and it was time to either try for baby number two or look into more long-term contraception options, like the implant.

We discussed it in depth and finally agreed that the time was right to try for a second child.

Going off any form of contraception was a bonus in so many ways. The natural lubrication in my vagina finally came back! Man, I was wetter than I'd ever been, and to add to that my libido had skyrocketed too. We were making crazy sexy love wherever and whenever we could. We were like two young lovers meeting for the first time.

It was no surprise we fell pregnant straight away again. We were fucking like rabbits when Ray was home on his week off, and Ray will tell you he has 'super sperm'.

WHERE DID THOSE NINE MONTHS GO?

It was the start of vintage at the winery when I fell pregnant. Forty-degree days spent out collecting wine samples—it was hard to hide the early signs of pregnancy. Again, I was lucky that morning sickness didn't come with vomiting, but it wasn't pleasant working a seven-day rotating roster completely exhausted. I couldn't even look at potato chips this time round but craved fast food fries and nibbled on nuts coated in salt during the worst times.

Being vintage time again and Ray working away, we had to come up with a solution for childcare. There was no way any facility would be able to accommodate the hours we needed. This is where my nan and pop came to the rescue. They cared for Brayden at their farm every week Ray was away. We would drive to meet them halfway in Renmark for pickups and drop-offs. If I got a weekend off, I'd go down and spend time with them and Brayden in between. It was hard to be away from Brayden for those extended periods of time, but I was glad he was spending quality time with family when he was away from me. I am forever grateful for how my grandparents helped us through that vintage. We would've been up shit creek without a paddle without them.

Vintage was over before I knew it, and I had made it through with the worst of the first trimester over. Even though doctors were concerned I may have problems with my cervix after my first pregnancy, after constant monitoring early on it was clear that my cervix was thick and healthy this time and ready to hold on to this baby until the very end.

Working full time was costing me more in childcare then it was worth, so I put in a request to go permanent part-time dayshift. Thankfully it was granted, and it gave me time to build my makeup business on the side. I was mainly going to clients' houses for bookings, but I had recently purchased a spray-tan machine and was offering tans from home, and I decided to set up the spare room to be able to do makeup from home too. I was busy, but I loved both jobs.

My second pregnancy was nearly textbook of my first (minus the complications), and I was convinced from the start that it was another boy. Again, we left it to be a surprise.

The time was getting near to my due date, and I was constantly on Ray to be looking for a job back home. His enthusiasm was less than desirable. I knew he was happy with his job now, but it just wasn't going to work for us once a second baby was on the scene. I was on his case persistently on the weeks he was home to go to the recruitment agencies and apply for anything and everything, but he was so fussy and stubborn, and he wasn't giving up his current job for just anything.

Thankfully, on a day he had decided to visit one of the agencies, a guy had called looking for someone to run his sand mine just twenty minutes from ours. He gave the guy a call, and the rest is history. He returned home before the birth and started his new job a week after.

THERE'S NO PLACE LIKE HOME

I forced myself to get out of the house as much as possible on days I felt really down during my second pregnancy, even if it was just a stroll along the river with B. It was hard but I knew it was best to get out into the fresh air instead of hiding inside of my dark mind.

I visited my best friend in Adelaide, with Brayden in tow, to escape reality during those times. I couldn't wait to hang out with her, chat and just relax. But I couldn't relax as hoped, being out of my comfort zone. I was out of the cosiness of my safe little home where everything was familiar and I could detach from the world. Now I was out in the suffocating world with no protection, and the need to just turn around and go home was overbearing.

I spent only two of the planned three days at her home. B and I camped out on a mattress in the lounge, and he still wasn't the best sleeper, whereas my bestie's son had slept through from day dot, so the pressure to keep Brayden quiet and not feel like we were a burden or keeping anyone awake in the house had me on edge so much so that I hardly slept a wink. My closest friend—a mother who had it all together, with the well-sleeping child—was making me feel more insecure and inadequate as a mother by the minute, but from no fault of her own. Why was I comparing myself so harshly to someone so close and dear to me?

Her husband was due to be back for the last night we were to stay. My girlfriend mentioned he had never lost a night of sleep since their son had come into the world, and instantly warning alarms started ringing in my ears. How could I guarantee my child wouldn't have a restless night and keep him awake the night before he was due to go back to work? I couldn't, and the inability to control the situation made me so sick to the stomach that it forced me to pack our bags and leave abruptly to head home. It was late in the day to leave, but I just knew I wouldn't survive another night there without having a major meltdown. I needed the safety cocoon of my own home. I felt terrible when I left and I just couldn't put into words to her at the time why it was that I just needed to go home.

It wasn't until my best friend read this book that she realised I was suffering immensely at that time. She felt I was quiet and a bit withdrawn during the visit, but she was none the wiser that on the inside I was in a constant battle with my mind.

HYPNO-BIRTHING

After Brayden's delivery I was convinced there was a more pleasant way to give birth, and I was right. A friend introduced me to the idea of hypno-birthing. Not having any idea of what hypno-birthing was, I started to do some research and I thought it was worth a shot. Ray took a bit of convincing, thinking it was some sort of hippie thing, but I was grateful when he finally chose to support my choice to do the course with me.

The first time I called Cyndi Power from the Power of Birth, I loved her instantly. Her bubbly personality oozed through the phone receiver, and I just knew I was going to be in safe hands. I explained that my husband worked away, and we weren't able to attend the set classes, and Cyndi was more than accommodating to fit us into a 1:1 full-day session, as this wasn't our first rodeo and we knew the basics of giving birth.

The day we spent with Cyndi was so informative, and Ray was great from the beginning and didn't hesitate when he was needed to participate. I left that room filled to the brim with knowledge and feeling more confident than ever about our upcoming birth.

WILL THIS BABY EVER COME OUT?

I took leave from the winery from thirty-six weeks pregnant, thinking I'd have an early baby again because, you know, each pregnancy is identical . . . clearly not the case. I kept doing tans and makeup jobs right up until the day before I went into labour. I had completely spring-cleaned my entire house from head to toe, including going through every single cupboard in the house after just the first week of leave.

The week's kept ticking by, and this baby had no plans on moving earth-side anytime soon. I had weekly check-ups with my obstetrician, and bub was still healthy and happy inside, so I was ready and willing to let nature take its course.

By forty weeks the obstetrician started to suggest a 'stretch and sweep'—a membrane adjustment to induce labour—but friends had told me horror stories about this process, and I was going to avoid it until it was a last resort. At forty weeks and five days, I was booked in for a stretch and sweep in two days. I contacted Cyndi, and she invited me straight over to her remarkable home on the riverbank to do a 'coming of the baby' session the following day. It was a beautiful experience, and I really felt it helped when it came to bringing the baby on naturally.

That evening I noticed I hadn't had any movement from the baby for what felt like hours. I did all the usual tricks to try to get a response, but nothing. I started to worry and expressed my concern to Ray. The typical response: 'Don't stress, babe, wait until the morning', but I knew I wouldn't sleep a wink until this baby moved, and I needed to reserve my rest as much as possible with the labour only around the corner. Brayden was already down for the night, so I decided I'd drive myself to the hospital, and Ray could stay home to care for Brayden. I made sure Ash was aware I was going to the hospital, so that if anything was to come of it she was ready for us to drop Brayden off in the middle of the night.

I arrived at the emergency department and explained my situation. I was assured a midwife would be down soon to escort me to the maternity ward. An hour later and I was still sitting there waiting, and the baby decided to start having a party in my womb. What a relief. I returned to the reception and suggested that I might just go back home as I have movement again, but they convinced me to stay and get it checked out just in case. Five minutes later, a midwife appeared to take me to the ward. They lay me on my back and attached the monitor to my stomach. The nurse advised me she would leave this on for twenty minutes and then return to review the results. As I lay there I could feel a discomfort in my back, and the baby was hosting a silent disco in there. The nurse returned to inform me not to worry, as the baby was well and there were contractions present, but they had to wait for the disco to finish before they could send me home, because there is now *too much* movement. After the twenty minutes was up, the nurse came back in with good news that I could head home, but she was sure she'd see me again in the early hours of the morning. I crawled into bed at twelve thirty a.m.

IT'S SHOWTIME

I drifted in and out of sleep for the next few hours before I got up at five thirty to pee. I was walking back to the bedroom when I got the familiar feeling of a slight amount of warm fluid running into my undies. Again, no waterfalls, like the movies, but I knew from past experience that shit was going to get real, and quick! After having such a rapid first labour, a few people jokingly said I might not make it to the hospital this time, and we did live twenty minutes away from the hospital now.

I casually let Ray know that things were starting to progress, and I checked in with Ash to let her know we'd drop Brayden off on the way to the hospital. I decided to have a shower and wash my hair, then blow-dry and straighten it. I don't know why I felt the need to do this on the morning I was in labour, but by the time I got to the straightening part, the contractions were closer and stronger than ever. I quickly called Ash to inform her we were going straight to Plan B: we weren't going to have time to stop on the way. She needed to come and pick Brayden up immediately. In the fifteen minutes it took her to arrive we had packed the bags into the car, and I was being stopped in my tracks with every contraction. I climbed into the passenger seat, kneeling and facing the wrong way, hugging the seat. Ray questioned my choice of positioning and the fact I didn't have a seatbelt on, but demon-possessed Penni was already rearing her ugly horns: '*I'm not turning around or putting my seatbelt on. I don't give a fuck—just drive, and fast!'*

Luckily it was in the early hours of the morning, and we didn't see a car on the road. I don't know how fast Ray drove, but I think we were both lucky we didn't run into any police along the way. When we pulled up at the hospital I was in mid-contraction, so Ray ran off into the hospital. At the time I was sure he had forgotten his wife in labour, and the bags in the car. The contraction passed and I thought to myself, *Where the fuck is he?* I proceeded to grab the bags out of the back and waddle towards the entry door. As I entered the building, Ray came along with a nurse and a wheelchair. Apparently, the nurses were having their morning meeting and he couldn't get anyone's attention any sooner. But we were there now and taken straight to the birthing suite. As soon as I entered the room, I collapsed to the floor on all fours, and demanded they give me the gas. There was no way anyone was going to change my mind and move me off that floor, even with their best efforts to get me onto the bed. They gave up and put a mattress on the floor for me to kneel on. Ray informed the midwives on duty that I had completed the hypno-birthing course and wanted as little interference as possible. Watching hypno-birthing videos, I witnessed women giving birth with no pain relief at all, and I bloody bow down to them. I had hoped to try, but fuck me, as soon as I got that gas into me I was a happy woman. The second experience on gas was better too. Firstly, I hadn't eaten myself stupid the night before and my thoughts went to happier places. Ray was fantastic, pushing my hips together throughout each contraction to relieve the pain, and man, did it help. He did complain about getting sore arms though, like a typical male. I was so much friendlier to the midwives this time round. I even asked a new one on duty how she was when she introduced herself to me. She was shocked that I was asking her when I was in the state I was. It became apparent not long after that we were heading into the last stage of the labour where you would traditionally push, but I wasn't going to this time. They removed my underwear and I began to follow my body's natural movements, just like I'd been taught in class. It honestly felt like I was doing the biggest shit of my life, on all fours. When I told Ray, he said, 'Babe, you did do a shit, and it had carrots in it.' Fuck, I couldn't stop laughing. I was worried Ray wouldn't be keen on doggie style after this experience, but thankfully it didn't tarnish his mind.

BABY NUMBER TWO

After only a short time in hospital, our second child was born at 7:40 a.m. Ray caught the baby and I asked if we had a little boy or girl. He said, 'A boy', and I felt my shoulders slump. Even though I had felt from the get-go it was a boy, being so stubborn and staying in until the last second made me think it could be a girl. But it was a stubborn little mini-Ray, and after I got over my minute of disappointment and rolled over to hold our son for the first time, I was more in love than ever. They say you never know if you can love your second child as much as your first, but you do. This little chubby bundle of joy stole my heart from the first second I laid eyes on him. It was a totally different feeling compared to the first time I held Brayden. We had two boys' names picked out, but we couldn't agree on a girl's name. Ray told me my suggestions were too old fashioned, and I felt his were names you'd only hear at your local strip club, so we were lucky it wasn't a girl. Straightaway I chose Hank out of the two names we had picked. I just knew it was the perfect name for him: Hank Ian, after my pop.

It's amazing to experience the difference between a baby being born at thirty-seven weeks and one at forty-one weeks. Brayden took time to open his eyes properly and suffered jaundice early on. Hank was wide-eyed and bushy-tailed from the moment he was born, and was even lifting his head up from Ray's chest that evening to suss him out.

BREAST OR BOTTLE SECOND TIME ROUND?

Leading up to the birth, I had already decided I wouldn't even contemplate breastfeeding the second time around. After the anxiety I felt after I had so much trouble with Brayden and that horrible hospital experience with mastitis, I just thought bub and I would be happier if we skipped the stress and went straight onto the bottle.

Hank was placed on my chest for the first time, and I couldn't help but draw him towards my breast to be able to hopefully feed on the colostrum milk. I still had no plans to feed past this point, but I knew how important these initial nutrients were for him.

Once we were taken to our room, Hank was showing signs of needing to feed. I had everything in place to bottle-feed, but the midwives were super busy at the time and we had no idea where to go to make up his formula. Ray suggested I try breastfeeding to settle him, but as soon as I tried to, the anxiety crept up my chest and all my past fears from Brayden came flooding back. I knew breastfeeding was not an option this time round.

Luckily, there was a lovely midwife on duty at the time. She entered the room moments later and asked if we were bottle- or breastfeeding. I felt instant relief! I said, 'Bottle', and showed her that I had everything packed in our hospital bag to be able to prepare the bottles. She assured me there was no need for that, and that she would go and prepare the bottle herself with the hospital supplies.

Unfortunately, Hank wasn't interested in the bottle at that time, but later on showed signs of wanting to feed again. The original bottle was cold and had sat for far too long, so I pressed the buzzer to get the attention of a midwife. A new midwife entered and asked what I needed. I asked if she could prepare a new bottle. She looked at me in utter disgust and replied, 'Why can't you prepare your own bottle? If you had planned to bottle-feed you should've been organised and bought everything you needed to the hospital.' At first I was in shock at her response; not because I expected her to wait on me hand and foot (I knew this wasn't a bloody five-star resort) but because she was the polar opposite of the previous nurse we had dealt with. When I explained to her through gritted teeth that I had everything I needed to be able to prepare bottles for my newborn child right here, and that I had only asked for her assistance due to the help we had received from the previous midwife, she obligingly showed me where the kitchen was. It was then that I asked what the minimum time I had to stay in hospital after a natural, no-complications birth was and then requested to be checked out immediately. It took them three hours to get everything sorted for us to be able to go home that night. The last thing we needed was for Hank to have done his first poo when they did his final checks. Thank the Lord there was that little tar-like poo in his nappy. Yes, my boy, we are going home, baby. We got home at eleven p.m. It was a long day, to say the least, but to curl up in the comfort of my own bed, surrounded by family, was the best end to the day I could've ever dreamed of.

ONE BABY IS NEVER LIKE ANOTHER

Hank initially started out in his bassinet in our room, but I found myself sneaking him into our bed from early on. There is just something about babies needing that close connection that I could never ignore, plus the bonus that we got longer stints between feeds. Ray was adamant that he didn't want another child that took up more room in our queen-size bed, so at three months, when I returned to work, I followed a controlled sleeping routine a close friend had passed on to me to try to get Hanky to self-settle. It was a long first night, sitting up and listening for the different types of cries, resettling him, and trying my absolute hardest to not just scoop him up and cuddle him in our bed again. It only took one very long night to get him to self-settle, though. From that night onwards, he was a dream to put to sleep at night. It was the polar opposite of the constant rocking and shushing we had to do with Brayden for so long. Even on nights when Hank would wake super upset, I'd try to pop him in with us, but he didn't want a bar of it. He preferred to have a quick cuddle and be placed back into his own cot. Even though it was a refreshing change to have a self-settling baby, I missed that closeness and felt slightly rejected in some way that Hank didn't need me like Brayden had. It wasn't until Hank was around one year old that he did a complete flip and wanted night-time cuddles. I don't know if it's because he missed out on cuddles for so long, but he is the biggest cuddlebug now, and we rarely get a night that one of us doesn't need to jump back in bed with him halfway through the night for cuddles. He grabs your arm and pulls it around him, demanding cuddles—it's so bloody cute. These days, we have a super-king-size bed that is seriously three adults wide, and the whole family can fit in without a hassle, much to my husband's dismay.

The other real difference between the two boys when they were young is the use of a dummy. I gave a dummy to both boys from early on to help with settling. Who knows what we would've done without one for Brayden for the first six months—it was the only thing that gave us some sort of relief from the crying. It was once Hanky was born that I was still trying to remove the dummy from Brayden's life; "ta-dum" he called it. Even though it was mainly for settling at home, I was at the point where enough was enough. I remember how much of a nuisance the dummy was in Brayden's early days when he was completely wrapped up, because every time he spat it during the night, we'd pop it back in for him before he'd settle again. I knew if Hank continued to have a dummy there would be no way he would learn to self-settle. I thought, *That's it, I'm going to remove all dummies from the house.* Hanky was none the wiser, but with Brayden I had to be a bit more cunning. I cut the end of the dummy off with scissors and threw it outside with the dog. I then proceeded to tell him a story of how the dog must've stolen his ta-dum. He was shattered and oblivious to the fact that he had more than one dummy, but it was the extreme measure I had to go to remove the dummy from his settling routine. We had some long nights following that day, but after a week ta-dum rarely got mentioned, unless it was to tell people the story of how his dog had eaten his dummy.

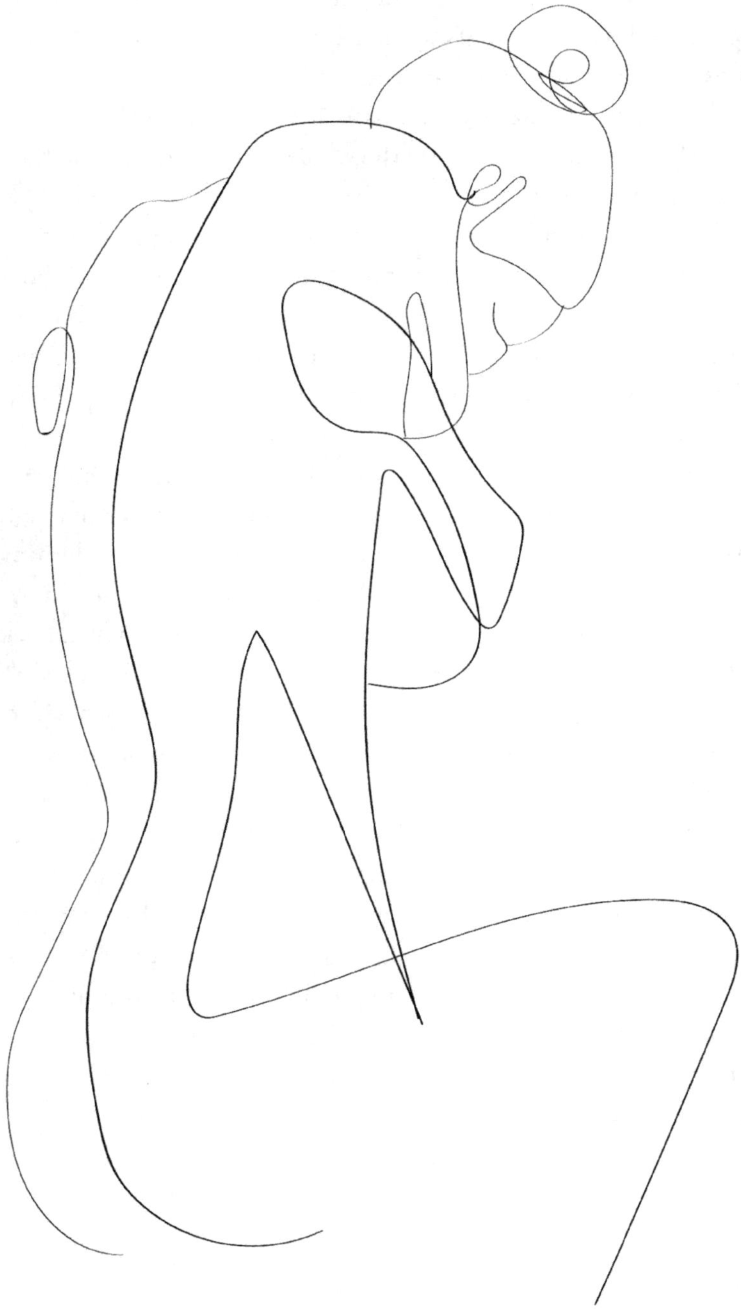

PART III

Mental Health

LIFE AS NORMAL

The first month seemed to go well with Hanky in our lives. We were still in the newborn bubble and he was thankfully different to Brayden as a baby, so the anxiousness of having another screaming baby twenty-four/seven was starting to ease. Leading up to the birth, everyone would say to me that it was unlikely I would have two very difficult newborns, but I wasn't going to cross out that possibility. In a way, I had started to convince myself that everything was going to be a breeze the second time round. But when the newborn-bubble burst and the sleep deprivation started to kick in, so did the reality of being home full time with two young children.

Even though I put in for six months maternity leave from the winery, I started working from home days after Hank was born. The beauty of doing makeup and tanning was that it slotted in well with Ray having weekends off. I always had trouble saying no to clients. I had worked so hard to build up my little business over the previous year that I hated letting any business go. I wish I knew then how much damage I was doing to my mental health by being busy all the time and overcommitting.

I knew I was starting to really struggle when Hank was about a month or so old. The stress of getting two kids ready to make it to appointments on time sent me into a major meltdown. The only time I felt like I had my shit together was when I was at a makeup job. It somehow gave me the escape I needed from what my everyday life had become. I was hanging out for my six weeks' post-birth clearance to be able to train again, because I was relying on it so much to help me to keep it together mentally.

I had a mums' night out at the movies in the midst of the world tumbling down on me. It was a fundraiser to see *Tully* starring Charlize Theron. For anyone who hasn't seen it, it was pretty much my life at that time on the big screen, playing before my eyes. It's a movie about a mother suffering from mental health who had imagined she had hired a night nurse to help her manage motherhood, and how clueless her husband had been about the whole thing. It is a very touching movie. After it finished, the women seated in front of us stood up and started to give their reviews. They commented that it was "OK," implying that it wasn't a showstopper by any means, and that they definitely wouldn't watch it again. I had my head bowed, trying to cover my tears. Those women were lucky because they couldn't relate to the main character. That character was me and it hit home, hard. I burst into tears when recounting this story to my mothers' group sitting with me. They knew I had been going through a tough time, and I think it was clearer now just how hard I was finding it to cope.

The early sign of my anxiety then was anger—uncontrollable anger. I didn't want to hurt my children in any way, but I needed to let off a bit of steam. If the kids were both screaming at me non-stop I'd remove myself from where they were and slam a door continually, or even punch it. Once, I slammed the back gate continuously, so hard that the lock broke off. Ray came home and asked me what had happened to the gate. I was honest and told him that I had slammed it so hard continuously that I had broken it. He looked at me, said no more and walked off. Not once did he ask if I was OK.

Frustration came part and parcel with the anger, and I was becoming a ticking time bomb if any tiny little thing didn't go to plan. I would swear and blame myself if I spilt something or I struggled to get the kids' belt buckles clipped in. Everyday tasks that sometimes took that slight bit more patience were becoming excruciatingly difficult to complete without blaming myself for fucking up all the time.

I NEED HELP

It was at my six-week post-birth check-up that I broke down to my obstetrician. I blurted out my feelings, the uncontrollable anger and frustration, everything. She suggested I see a counsellor immediately.

I started seeing a counsellor who bulk-billed for new mums for the first year of their baby's life. And at the start, it really felt like it was helping to get everything off my chest by talking to someone who had the time to listen without judgement. My mum friends were all so busy then. Most of us had returned to work or even had a second child to care for, and I didn't want to bother others with my burdens. I guess I was putting on a brave front, not wanting people to know the monster I had become or the fact that I wasn't the supermum they all believed me to be.

One thing I should've got from those initial sessions was that I was over-committing myself big time, and I needed to slow down. The one thing that I was taking away was that I was holding all the pressure of our family on my shoulders and it was only a matter of time before I collapsed.

I started to go back to the gym, and it was my nonnegotiable with Ray, that one hour a day to myself to grunt and sweat out the stress. It made me feel a thousand times better, mentally.

But when Hank was only three months old, instead of slowing down I returned to the winery from maternity leave early, at the start of vintage, working full time and rotating between afternoon- and nightshift.

I was so lucky to have such an understanding boss to accommodate the flexibility I needed to return to work and still care for my children, as we needed the money. Ray and I had discussed this before Hank was born and I had expressed that I didn't want to be rushed back to work again. I wanted it to be my decision . . . when I was ready. Maybe I just didn't have what it took to be a stay-at-home mum?

I went into autopilot once I returned to work. I look back now and I still don't know how I lasted the vintage. On nightshift, I would care for the boys during the day, try to get a nap in when they did, and once Ray returned home from work I'd try to get a solid three to five hours' sleep, if I was lucky, before I went back again. I've always been a hard worker. No matter what occupation I've had, my work ethic never changes. And at this time it was no different; if anything, I was even more determined and focused because I was doing it for my family's survival.

Those three to four months of vintage went by like a blur, and before I knew it I made it out the other end—alive, but utterly exhausted. I hadn't been able to maintain any kind of physical exercise with the demands of my work roster, and my mental health was diminishing by the day. I was still putting on a front to the outside world, including family and friends, as well as keeping up with my rapidly growing makeup business.

During this time, it was when I was home alone with the boys that my anxiety got the better of me. Keeping a brave face on to the outside world was tiring. I would screen phone calls and never reply to messages, even if they were from my closest family and friends, and hide away through the feeds of social media. I opened up to my best friend, but not even she understood the depth I was in with my mental health (until later). Maybe it was because I never spoke about it like it was a big deal, trying to make light of it at the time.

I kept seeing the counsellor, and it was helping me to talk aloud about the week I'd struggled through, but I was definitely going downhill, and fast. Life had caught up with me, and it was about to bite me on the arse—hard!

And this now brings us back to the start of the book, when anxiety was a real bitch—and still is.

When I was seeing the counsellor at this time, we spoke about the assistance of medication to help me out of the hole I had dug myself into. I don't know why I was so against it at the time. I was probably worried about judgement from family, friends, even complete strangers. I thought I was strong enough to get out of it naturally with the aid of exercise, removing caffeine, etc. Maybe I just didn't want to admit I was weak at the time, that life had beaten me at that point.

The thing that made it harder was the counsellor never said that I needed to get a script for anti-anxiety medication, that I was a screw loose from crazy and it was time to get medicated help. So it was left up to me. But no-one wants to admit they've lost the fucking plot—you want someone else to point that out to you. You tend to listen more when it comes from the outside, someone who specialises in this shit. I knew I was going crazy, but just how crazy? Was I borderline crazy? Or was I a step away from a loony bin? I needed her to tell me that. But she never did, so it took until I painted the kitchen walls with our family roast dinner to tell her that I needed medication.

I saw our family doctor straight after my appointment with her. I was so embarrassed. He was probably a similar age to Ray and me; he had a young child too and was the best family doctor we have ever had. He was thorough and knew his shit. Of course, there was no judgement from his end, and he prescribed a suitable medication.

While I was coming to terms with my own diminishment of mental health, I was also dealing with Ray's. Trying to get a man to admit something is wrong and that he needs help is a hard task.

Getting him to a doctor for help was even harder. Ray had turned into a ticking time bomb too; his motivation had diminished and our house had turned into a living hell. We were both living on eggshells and we could hardly stand each other. Every day was a game of who was more tired, did more around the house, worked harder . . . and the list went on. It was not healthy.

Thankfully, he came to terms with the fact that neither of us were the people we used to be, and it was no longer healthy to continue without seeking professional help. We saw our family doctor together, and I was really surprised by how honest and open Ray was with him. Even Ray commented afterwards how good it was to get things off his chest. Us girls, we love to talk about everything and anything, and I think we forget how lucky we are to have the ability to do it so freely, to be able to open up about our emotions with ease. Men bottle everything up! It's not natural for them to go to the pub and spill their emotions to their mates over a schooner; traditionally it can be seen as a weakness to not be able to cope with life, to be seen as being weak in the mind. Could you imagine bottling everything up? How suffocating that would feel? So, this appointment was huge progress for our family, and I was super proud of him.

TIME FOR A CHANGE

After a month or so back at work part time, I was starting to really dislike working at the winery. I'm not sure exactly what it was, but I knew I needed a change. I felt that if work was my three days to escape motherhood, I wanted to be doing something that I loved.

I had a hair appointment during this time of uncertainty, and it was then that I made up my mind to return to beauty therapy, a job that didn't pay as much as the winery but was something I loved and missed doing. The salon in which my hairdresser worked was searching for a beauty therapist to try to build the beauty side of their business. *Perfect*, I thought.

Once I met the salon owner for an interview, I felt an instant fire light up in my belly. This was the right place for me at that time. We hit it off straight away: both working mums with young children and a passion for our industries and business.

Treating clients again was like therapy for me. I loved skincare and facial treatments the most, but just to be able to make others feel relaxed and good about themselves was so rewarding. Being a business that was in the growing stage when it came to the beauty side, I had the pressure of trying to build the clientele as well as treating them. Some days I loved the challenge, other days I felt like it pushed my anxiety through the roof because I didn't want to fail. Not just for my own ego, but for the business. I truly felt the potential was there.

DO WHAT YOU LOVE

I had done my diploma in beauty therapy straight out of school, followed by my diploma in makeup in my early twenties. I spent four years in Melbourne, managing a chain of high-end luxury cosmetic stores before I made the life-changing decision to move to Kalgoorlie. I love the art of makeup, and the fact that the majority of work is done on weekends makes it easier to work around a young family.

When I started doing a bit of makeup again when Brayden was young it was more of a hobby to start off with, a little extra income but also a way to let my creative juices flow. I started doing a few odd jobs here and there, and then it slowly started to build up by word of mouth. I began to do online masterclasses with other makeup artists who I found inspirational to update my skills and techniques.

I felt like I had to move my business to a more central location for clients to be able to build it up to the next level. I found a local salon that didn't offer makeup and I rented a chair there on Saturdays.

It wasn't until I did my first local wedding that my business really started to blossom. You can have a portfolio of photos of previous weddings you have done, but in a country town you need to do a local wedding, and do it well, for word of mouth to become your greatest form of advertisement.

I loved doing makeup for the transformations, and not always in a dramatic way, either. My style of makeup has always been to highlight someone's natural beauty. I wasn't big on caking on layers of foundation.

It was a wedding that I did in August 2018 that cemented to me that I did this for the joy I could bring to others, not the money.

I hadn't met the bride until the day of her wedding, which made me super nervous, because brides are generally quite specific in the look they want on their big day. I like to do a trial prior so I know I will nail the look for them. We communicated a few times over Messenger only a few months before the date. I did encourage a trial, but she said she wouldn't have the time as she was in and out of hospital. I didn't think much of it, presuming a family member was unwell or that she worked in a hospital. It wasn't until I arrived on the day, when the beautiful bride-to-be answered the door and I noticed her bald head and the oxygen bottle beside her, that I realised she was unwell. I nearly burst into tears on the spot. She was the most down-to-earth person I had ever met, and I just wanted to ask the man above, *Why her? She has two young girls, a loving partner, and their whole life ahead of them, why take her?* The diagnosis was quick and final, so their wedding had been brought forward to this date so they could marry before she was taken too early. She had lost all her hair, including her eyebrows. This was the most important face I had ever transformed. It was up to me to bring back the youth and life that had been stripped from this beautiful woman's face. It was up to me to bring tears to her eyes when she looked in the mirror and saw a glimpse of her former self before disease took it all from her. I held back tears when I did her makeup that day (I'm crying now as I relive it). She was so accepting of her fate. She had come to terms with what the future was to be for her, and she was OK with it now. She was one of the bravest people I have ever met. After I finished her makeup, she put on her gorgeous long and flowing rose-gold wig and looked at her reflection in the mirror. Her response was the reason why I love doing what I do, even if I don't make a bloody dime for it. She was the most beautiful bride, and if you didn't know her you would have never known the torture she was living through on the inside that day.

I would check her social media for months after the wedding, hoping for some miracle to occur and that she was going to be able to watch those beautiful girls of hers grow up. Unfortunately, that miracle never came, and I learned from a mutual friend who had posted on social media that she had sadly passed away. I bawled my eyes out when she told me. I'm sobbing now. I can't describe the honour I feel that she trusted me on that day to be a part of one of her last, most precious memories. Life can be cruel sometimes, and ever so short.

A CHANGE IS AS GOOD AS A HOLIDAY

The salon was going well and my business was booming, even though financially I wasn't making much. My salon income was luckily just enough to cover childcare and my fuel to work and back. The medication was starting to level out my anxiety and Ray wasn't as angry anymore. We started to see a couple's counsellor to try to break down the wall of resentment that had been building up between us over time, and it did help, initially, even if it was to just have a civil conversation between the two of us. At the end of the sessions we were required to say one thing we loved about each other, but it couldn't be the same. This was the best part of the session, because I never felt like Ray loved or appreciated anything about me, seeing as he never said or showed it. Learning that he did appreciate all I did for us was nice to finally hear aloud.

We started drinking more on weekends, and just spent time at home when not working. Ray started to dislike his job, so we spent days trying to work out what he wanted to do. He wasn't happy just to do any old thing, and if he wasn't happy in his job it made life harder for the rest of the household.

One Sunday afternoon we were out in the backyard with the kids, smashing a carton. A job for mining in the Hunter Valley arrived in Ray's inbox and he showed it to me. We discussed how good it would be to get back into mining for the roster and income. We had looked at the Hunter Valley as an option to move to when returning from WA to start a family, but were against it because it was so far away from family. The funny thing is we were the ones doing majority of the traveling from Mildura to visit family. They rarely came to visit us.

Now, anyone who knows me well knows that if I'm determined about something, I'll do everything to make it happen. And the decision to move interstate was no different.

From that day, I updated both our resumes and contacted several different recruitment agencies in the Hunter region with ads on online recruitment sites at the time. I spoke to them personally, emailed our resumes, and then followed up with them again to make sure they had received them. I didn't hear back from the one ad that had caught our eye initially, but the second one I contacted got back to us within a day. The staff were so helpful and friendly, and we got the ball rolling straight away with interviews.

The next step was to sell our house. We already had the Kalgoorlie property that cost us an arm and a leg to keep as a so-called 'investment', so there was no way we wanted the drama of a second. We had only owned the house for a couple of years, so we knew there wouldn't have been much of a change in the value; we were happy to just get back what we paid for it. If we went through a real estate agent, there was no way we'd get back much with the cost of fees. The neighbour knew we were thinking of selling and had a mate over one night who had been looking for a house but just couldn't get a break in the market, as houses sold quickly in town and generally in the first round of offers. He drove to our place and introduced himself and his partner—the rest is history, as they say. We couldn't have asked for fate to be any more on our side that day.

I had now secured us jobs and our current house was in the contract stage, so I now had to find us a new home in NSW. Neither Ray nor I had spent any time in the state, so we had no idea what to expect or where to live. I searched online for the closest towns and narrowed down a few affordable places. Now, if Ray and I were going to go back to full-time work on the same roster, we would need someone to care for the boys. I had looked into the option of hiring a nanny locally, and it seemed like it could be an option initially but quite costly long-term, since we would require them to stay overnight when we were doing nightshifts. I started to sign up for au-pair websites, as I thought this could be the most affordable way to go. I had heard of good and bad experiences. It was hit and miss, and when Ray's mates got wind of it—putting their two bob in about having an attractive young girl around the house—I just thought that this wasn't the right option for us. Not because I didn't trust Ray, but because I personally wanted someone with childcare experience so I could work shifts and be assured that my kids were in good hands, not just eye candy for my husband and mates who was purely in the country for the cultural experience and not my children's welfare. I also wanted it to be a long-term position, and au pairs are limited in the time they can stay with one family. I had no idea where to start, so I got online, searching companies that assist in finding the perfect nanny for your situation. The boys were still young at the time, and I didn't want to trust them with just anyone. I wanted experience. I found a Brisbane-based company that assisted with all types of childcare, from short- to long-term. They were helpful from the get-go, and after writing a small story about our family, they agreed that we were in search of a live-in nanny to suit our requirements. They came back promptly with a candidate, and after a phone call with the potential nanny we knew she was the perfect fit for our family. She is still with our family two years later.

Having a live-in nanny now on board changed our rental requirements, and I was trying to find a place with separate living accommodations for her, so she would be able to get a break from the family on her days off due to our lifestyle roster. There was nothing until the day before Ray was due to drive over for the inspections, when a lovely house on an acre block with a separate granny flat and massive shed popped into my inbox. I knew this had to be our new home! I showed Ray and he was sceptical, because it was thirty minutes from our mine site, but it was more like the country living we were used to, not fence-to-fence with neighbours in a new housing estate with driveways steeper then Mount Everest.

Ray viewed all the properties, and he fell in love with the one out in the small country town of Jerrys Plains. Luckily, the owner was at the property to show him through and they hit it off like a house on fire. He called me as soon as he left and said, "This is the one." I was straight onto the computer to apply online. I then called to make sure they had received the application. The agent had only just got back into the office from the property and was blown away by how efficient I was at getting the application in. They forwarded our application to the owner, who was happy to sign the rental agreement over to us.

Last but not least was getting everything moved. I booked a removalist to move the bulky items and we loaded up two cars, the trailer, and the boat with the rest of our belongings. My grandparents had the boys whilst we drove over for the first time. We thought it best if we set everything up and did our final medicals without the boys in tow. We did have one cat on board, though. The second had gone MIA the day we were due to leave, so we would have to go back and find her when we grabbed the kids. After a very busy couple of days of unpacking and finding our bearings, we were back on the road to pick the boys and the second cat up and show them our new home. Luckily, the new house owners of our old place were able to catch our runaway cat whilst we were moving so we had all the family ready to go. Plus, my niece's girlfriend had agreed to come and care for the boys for the first couple of weeks until the nanny finished up at her current family and moved over. She was an absolute lifesaver! It was a long, cosy fourteen-hour drive over, but we made it in one piece, and the boys loved the new place straight away.

It took three months from that Sunday when we first looked at that job advertisement to have our whole family uplifted interstate for a new beginning. Did it take its toll on me mentally? Of course it did. I increased my medication in the early days of the move because the tell-tale signs were there that my anxiety was going to increase immensely with the stress that was about to be put on me.

WORK-LIFE BALANCE

Choosing to move interstate was the best decision we could have ever made. We dug ourselves out of a financial hole and removed ourselves from the toxic environment that our home had become due to the stress of it. I never minded mining before, but for me the choice to return was more about the balance it would bring to our lives.

The hardest part about moving from Mildura was leaving my business behind. I had worked so hard and sacrificed so much for it. I had a few weddings booked in for the first six months I had moved away, and I returned to honour them. There was no way I was going to let my beautiful brides down.

Returning to mining meant that Ray and I could both work full time but also have the same time off with the boys. I can't say driving huge dump trucks is an exciting job, but I definitely feel lucky to have had the opportunity to return to the lucrative industry of mining. The most important aspect of the job was that the roster we were going to be on meant we would have just as much time off as we worked. In the space of four weeks we worked seven dayshifts, seven nightshifts, and had fourteen days off: the perfect work-life balance, and that was our number-one priority.

Sometimes it's not just the type of job that gives you work satisfaction. It can be the perks of the job, and the freedom it brings to your life.

MONEY CAN'T BUY HAPPINESS

Ray and I have had ongoing conversations about the effects that money has on a relationship, and on a person's happiness overall. Now, don't get me wrong, I am well aware that financial struggle is high on the list when it comes to marital issues, but it isn't the answer for marital bliss, either.

Moving interstate was a fresh start, and yes, we were finally going to be able to be more comfortable financially. However, the honeymoon period of the move would soon be over and the cracks in our marriage would once again resurface.

In the first year in NSW, we paid off debt, spent money on things we hadn't been able to afford since having the kids, and, most importantly, we had someone to care for the boys so we could finally get some time together as a couple. We went on date nights, music festivals at vineyard with friends, weekends away, and finally got to enjoy each other's company without the stress of the kids surrounding us. Our relationship really did do a complete flip and I started to fall back in love again. We have always loved each other, but I believe you fall in and out of love throughout a marriage, and it was so nice to fall back in love again.

I think that when you keep yourself super busy you tend to oversee the issues surrounding you at the time. We had such a hectic and social first year, and everything was so new and exciting, that we were too busy to see that the cracks we had temporarily glued back together when we initially moved were starting to come apart again.

Because I was feeling so good when we first moved, I thought I should reduce my dose of medication back to the original amount. I slowly reduced it over time, as the doctor had recommended, and it wasn't until about a month of the reduced amount that I found my signs of anxiety increase massively—the anger, the inability to cope with everyday things. Ray noticed too and spoke up, so I went straight back to the doctor to resume an increased dosage. At the same time, I had noticed an increase in Ray's anger and lack of motivation since the stress of the move. I brought it up multiple times that I thought he should see the doctor to reassess his dosage, but he just kept putting it in the too-hard basket; it wasn't until eighteen months later that I would finally get him to go and get his medication reassessed. Living with someone who has a short fuse, with everything coming out of their mouth in frustration and anger, is very taxing on everyone in that household. It's not pleasant at all. It's not only you who is living with a mental illness, it's your family too, and if you don't like how you are reacting to things, how do you think your family feels having to live with that every day? It's so common these days, but it is such a tough subject for people to talk about openly, or to reach out for help about, rather than putting on a brave face for the outside world. Ray is a completely different person at work than at home, and workmates always seem surprised if the topic of his short fuse at home is discussed. I get frustrated with Ray because I feel I have to do so much for him, otherwise he just doesn't get it done. Keeping a check on his mental health, and carefully picking the time to bring up certain subjects, like revisiting the doctor, is taxing, but I'm glad that I do it, because I know how much harder it is for men to face these demons, especially on their own, and there's no way I'd risk losing him in the boys' or my life.

YOU'RE SO LUCKY YOUR HUSBAND CAN BABYSIT YOUR KIDS

This is a comment I get quite regularly that really gets under my skin. Firstly, a father does not 'babysit' his own kids. He cares for them, the same as a mother does. We are both as responsible as each other for the wellbeing of our children. I never wanted the father of my children to not know where the nappies were or how to care for his kids if I had to duck out for a bit. We are living in a generation now where it's not as common, or traditional, for dads to be the sole provider for the family, or for women to be stay-at-home mums. The times are a-changin' people, and why are women expected to take on the responsibility of working more to help provide for the family but men are not required to pick up the slack with the domestic duties?

I returned to work when Brayden was eight months old, as Ray's income couldn't support us, and then, when Hank was only three months, I returned to full-time shift work again for the same reason. This meant that Ray and I shared the responsibility of supporting our family. So, tell me why the responsibility at home shouldn't be shared?

Having bottle-fed the boys early on made it easier for Ray to be a more hands-on dad with both children. He'd had experience with his own nieces and nephew from an early age, and fatherhood came quite naturally to him.

Yes, I am lucky that my husband is a hands-on father and confident to care for the boys just as well as I do, but I don't believe it's a reason for the household responsibility to be left all up to me. I'm going to give you an example. Ray will look after the boys while I do the grocery shopping. When I return, there will be dishes and shit everywhere. So, within the first hour I'm home, I'm lugging in bags of groceries, putting it all away, and cleaning up the disaster that's been left for me. I can guarantee you that Ray does not have to do the same, nor would he come straight home and start tidying anything. He also doesn't have to think about whether there's going to be another toilet roll in the bathroom cupboard when he uses the last one, what the kids will eat for the week, what he'll eat for the week, if his phone bill will be paid on time, can we afford groceries this week . . . and the list goes on. A mother's/wife's/woman's mind is working on overdrive from the minute she wakes up to the minute she can finally switch her mind off when she goes to bed. Add some anxiety into the mix and you are also overthinking everything else in your life in between the important stuff.

Ray and I now work equally with the same amount of time off. Friends feel I should give him a break because 'at least he can look after the kids.' They wish their husbands could do the same and that I should take the good with the bad, but I still don't feel like this is fair. My anxiety tells me it isn't fair that I'm running around like a blue arse fly while he's sitting back on the couch or burying his head in his phone. Many hands make light work, and if we hooked into it all together then maybe we could both be sitting on the couch, relaxing.

The most important thing I've learnt from couples counselling is not to play the comparison game, which is the hardest thing not to do in a marriage. Who does more? It gets worse when children come into play. You each think you are doing more than the other. And women, let's be honest: we generally bloody are! But it takes a conscious effort to not sit there running a list in your head of the hundred things you've done so far, compared to the one thing your husband had to do but still needed reminding about. It's frustrating as fuck. I still struggle every day to remove these thoughts because they only make me more pissed off; they don't achieve anything. I've realised over time that my husband doesn't see the world like I do, nor does he excel in multitasking. A mum will walk through the house, turn off the TV that's been left on, pick up random toys from the ground, remove the washing out of the machine and hang it up. She'll walk past the chicken coop, feed the chooks and collect the eggs. She'll return inside, do the dishes left on the sink by everybody but herself, and then wonder why she was walking through the house in the first place. Your husband will walk that same route and will likely trip on those toys, swear about them being left in the way but won't pick them up, and continue on with his day. It's taken me years to drill into my head that my husband doesn't see what I see when walking around the house, so I can either stew on everything he doesn't do because he can't read my mind, or I could just ask him what I need him to help with—or I can just do it myself, because it's sometimes bloody quicker.

Marriage requires a lot of teamwork and consideration for each other. It is something you have to work on continually. Some days it flows, other days it's a complete shit fight.

WHEN DO YOU KNOW YOU'RE DONE?

Ray and I had said from the start that we only wanted two kids. Of course, everyone wants the pigeon pair, with a boy and a girl, and I was no different, but I always said that if I had two of the same sex, I'd rather two boys.

It wasn't until Ray had his vasectomy that I came to terms with the fact that I was done. Even in the weeks after his operation, I was considering whether we should try one last time, while there was still a slight chance it might work. I always imagined a little mini-me running around, and it took me a long time to accept that I wasn't going to have a daughter.

Now, I love my boys to death, but it didn't stop me craving a little girl. I was so clucky when it came to girls. I lost my mind in the girls' section of department stores when I saw the cuteness of their little outfits. Financially, it was probably safer that we didn't end up having a girl.

The counsellor I saw after the birth of Hank advised me not to have any more children, due to the instability of my mental health. She thought a third child would be the icing on the cake that tipped me over the edge, and for some time I agreed with her.

Once we moved interstate, I started thinking maybe I could cope with another child. I had help now, and we were financially stable. I think a huge part of the reason why I desired a third child was because it was my last chance to get it right, one more chance to prove to myself that I was a good mum and I could get through the newborn stage sane. Everything I did wrong the first two times I would do right this one. I would make up for all my mistakes!

When reflecting on the past five years, the one thing I know I did wrong was overcommit myself rather than slowing down and being present, enjoying the early years of motherhood. Maybe if I had taken a step back and slowed down it wouldn't have all gone to shit. Maybe if I decided to try for a little girl, with all my ducks in a row, I would just sit back and enjoy every minute of it. But it was all just maybes. There were no certainties, there never are in life, and it wasn't a gamble I was willing to take after finally feeling like life was getting back on track.

THE EFFECT MENTAL HEALTH CAN HAVE ON RELATIONSHIPS

Living in a home that has not only one but two parents suffering from mental health issues makes it a challenging environment to be in. I am very lucky that Ray has opened up to me and is open about getting help for mental illness. This doesn't make it any easier to live with, though.

Mental illness is an ongoing battle. You can take medication to assist with the symptoms of it, but it can flare back up at any time. It's about trying to find what triggers these flare-ups, and how to prevent them as much as possible.

I sometimes feel like it's a catch-22 for me. My anxiety gets bad when I'm running around trying to get everything done with no help from Ray, or having to ask Ray to do the simplest thing a thousand times before he'll actually do it, or I'll get so fed up I'll just do it myself, as it will be quicker with less hassle. But if there are some things I can't do that I need Ray to do, it's absolutely infuriating. I'm then worried about his mental health and blame that for his lack of motivation, poor short-term memory, etc. But I sometimes feel like Ray never considers how his actions affect my mental health.

I hate being late! I get so anxious if I'm running behind, which causes me to get angry and short with others around me at the time. Ray is forever causing us to run late. We'll already be late to leave and he'll just have to go and grab something, or he'll stay in the shower too long because he hasn't left himself enough time. Whatever the reason being, he seems to have no appreciation for the effect that running late has on my mental state, even though we have spoken about it before.

So, living in a house of cray-crays is hard work, wanting to do what's best for you but at the same time wanting to make sure it doesn't have a negative effect on the other.

The relationship that has been most affected by my anxiety is the close relationship I had with my nan. Before I moved interstate we used to speak weekly. She was someone I could talk to about anything, and I knew she supported me no matter what. I'd told her when I first started on medication for anxiety, and she knew all the ins and outs of my marriage. I felt as soon as I moved that our relationship changed somewhat. My nan has this tone that's hard to decipher when you are talking on the phone, and it always made my anxiety rise. Was she angry with me? She hardly called me anymore, as my roster was too confusing for her to work out when to call, so it was left up to me to make the call, and I was always nervous of the nan I was going to get on the other end. Eventually I stopped calling as much. I couldn't mentally deal with not knowing if I was going to get a happy nan, open for a good chitchat, or if it was going to be awkward and feel like I was trying to get water out of a rock. This was a horrible feeling, and in the end I had to choose between feeling nearly physically ill every time I got the courage to call her or take a step back. I love my nan to death and miss her, and the close relationship we had every day, but I couldn't mentally cope with what our relationship had become. We speak now and then, and I'm hoping one day it will be what it was before, but for now, anxiety wins.

THE BIG O

When I started writing this book, I hadn't had an orgasm during intercourse since Hank was born. Yep, ladies, you heard me right: that's two and a half years with no fireworks during sex. Not that I'm counting. Now, I've never been a woman who orgasmed easily through intercourse, and it definitely didn't happen every time, but with the help of battery-operated sex toys it was more times than less, so when I discovered it was actually impossible after Hank's arrival I thought I'd broken my vagina.

I got back on the horse a lot sooner after baby number two. I hadn't needed stitches the second time round and everything seemed to feel normal a lot sooner. I put that down to the second pregnancy and birth not being as traumatic as the first. I didn't have to recover as much internally and spiritually the second time round.

It wasn't until a few months post-birth that I picked up on the fact that it was not only impossible to orgasm during sex, but I couldn't even climax on my own, which had never been a problem before. I got the implant put in place for birth control at six weeks post-birth. As expected, I spotted for six weeks after, which I was informed was quite normal. I then had nothing, and sex returned to normal minus the fireworks.

It was approximately seven months after Hank was born that I started anxiety medication. One of the side effects of the medication can be lack of libido. Now, it wasn't that I didn't want to have sex, I did, but I bloody needed a mind-blowing orgasm at the end too!

It wasn't until I'd had the implantin for a year that I started to bleed heavily, and it wouldn't stop. It was coming up to three weeks of nonstop period when I decided that enough was enough. I booked an appointment with the doctor and demanded they remove it immediately. Ray and I had already spoken about him getting the snip, and this event had just cemented that this is the way we would go from then on with regards to our contraception.

The bleeding was more of a blessing in disguise than I knew at the time. Removing the hormones being pumped through my body made excess weight easier to lose and my natural lubrication come back. Sex was feeling great again, but unfortunately I still couldn't climax, no matter how hard and what we tried. I was, however, able to come again on my own, with a little help of some online movies to concentrate my mind.

The last time I visited the doctor to renew my anxiety medication script, I brought up the inability to be able to climax during sex. The doctor believed that the medication could have negative effects on the urge to want to have sex, not the ability to orgasm, so we left it at that. It wasn't until I started seeing a psychiatrist recently that I spoke of my frustration of not being able to get satisfaction during sex, and how it was affecting my sexual desire, because even though it was enjoyable, nearly three bloody years without that relief at the end was doing my head in. I felt like sex was just for Ray's pleasure these days. The psychiatrist explained that there may be a psychological reason why I couldn't climax, and she was spot on the money. That and a lack of foreplay, because we all know that with kids you don't have the pleasure of being able to jump each other whenever you like. You are usually on a short timer whilst the kids are distracted by their iPad, TV show or whatever other creative way you can come up with to fit in a quickie. In fact, a quickie soon ends up being the norm, and you can't remember the last time you spent more than five minutes in the act.

It seems so simple, now that I think about it. Women need to be so much more mentally prepared for sex than men. Men look at a naked body, or a set of tits, and they're as hard as a rock, raring and ready to go. Women, on the other hand, generally can't just look at an erect dick and instantly turn into a wet 'n' wild downstairs. A woman's orgasm is more like baking a cake: getting the right ingredients in place, carefully preparing them and then baking it for the perfect amount of time at the right temperature. I never considered that my overthinking from anxiety had affected me between the sheets. During sex, I was overthinking every little thing Ray was doing or even just about everything else that was going on at that time, and not just in the bedroom. I was also concentrating so hard on the end prize that the in-between stage just wasn't there. I'd have that pre-orgasm feeling arise, but then I'd think so hard about it that it would run away and hide. The psychiatrist told me to just focus on the sensations that were happening at the time, nothing else.

One morning after a nightshift, after we had had a shower quickie the night before, I couldn't wait to get home and jump him. I just kept thinking of Ray all night at work. I expressed to him in the car that he had been on my mind, and he was as eager as me to jump into bed without the kids interrupting us. We got home and showered, and I snuck off into the walk-in robe to put on a little sexy number I hadn't worn for him yet and jumped into bed. It was so good to feel our naked bodies against each other and to have the freedom to explore the foreplay that we hadn't done in ages. I kept my mind from wandering and concentrated only on the feel of Ray's kisses and tongue. Once we started to have sex, I came within minutes and it was the biggest relief ever. I had missed that slow build-up to absolute euphoria so much! It was like we had been building a wall between us for so long, and we finally made it come crashing down. Whether it was the build-up of the thought of it all night at work, the strength I've gained over my mind or the concentration of every little sensation, it worked, and I prayed it wasn't a once-off. The mind is such a powerful tool, and I believe the thoughts you put into the universe can, and, will happen.

THE MUM'S GUILT

Every mum out there knows what it feels like to have the mum's guilt, am I right? We experience this sickening feeling daily: guilty if we go to work; guilty if we lose our patience; guilty that we are doing something for ourselves even though we know it's a necessity to have some 'me time'; guilty that we are allowing our kids too much screen time, questioning how much is too much, but then guilty again if we deprive them of technology and how to operate it, as it will likely be a staple of school life for them in the future. And the list goes on and on. The role of being a mother is a selfless one. We give and give to make sure everyone around us is happy before considering ourselves. Why do we still experience this overwhelming feeling of guilt, then? I wish I knew the answer to this. However, I do prioritise 'me time', such as placing going to the gym higher up on my to-do list because I know it doesn't only benefit my state of mind, but also the mum and wife I am on a daily basis. I am currently in the middle of a '21-Day Change Your Mindset Challenge' offered online with Belinda Anderson. Belinda is based here in Australia and offers women's holistic wellness retreats in Australia, as well as Fiji and Bali in pre–COVID-19 days. The difference I have felt in such a short amount of time by consciously being aware, changing my thought patterns and learning to live in the now is astonishing. Before partaking in this challenge, I used to think of meditating as some sort of hippie ritual; I have now realised it is a game-changer. I have committed to daily meditation since commencing this experience and have been blown away by the mind's ability to slowly begin to consciously live in the now when trained how to. If you haven't tried it before, I highly recommend you jump online and treat yourself. There are thousands of different meditations available online My go-to channel is the Mindful Movement. I now follow a one-hour meditation in the evening when going to bed, focusing on relieving stress and anxiety in my life, and ten minutes before rising in the morning to concentrate on bringing gratitude and positivity into my day. To all the mums out there, give yourself a break! Mum-life is bloody hard; pour yourself a wine and look back on the day, proud that you got through it with everyone still alive and in one piece. Focus on what was great about the day, how you met any challenges head-on, what you learnt from them, and move on to bigger and better things the following day. But most importantly, remember to breathe and be kind to yourself.

NEGATIVITY BREEDS NEGATIVITY

I recently removed all the social media apps from my phone. I just had to go cold turkey on this shit and I was spending way too much time mindlessly scrolling through crap. The other issue I have when my anxiety is at its peak is OCD, and I can't handle any apps on my phone having any little red notification circles present. It drives me insane. Now don't get me wrong, I love a good social media filter. The big-mouth 'rant' filter was my fave, especially when you are doing exactly that, having a rant, usually about your husband or kids. But I was starting to live through my social media outlet more than being present in my real life.

It was initially twenty-one days that I promised myself I would remove the apps for; it has now been months and I still have not downloaded them back onto my phone. Friends have messaged, asking if I'm OK because I've been so quiet, and it made me realise how much I was sharing my life over a form of social media, because as soon as I disappeared off it, it became apparent that it was really the only way friends were keeping up with what was happening in my life.

After removing social media I came to understand how much negativity I was breeding inside myself and promoting outwards by the things I would share. We are all too familiar with the annoying things our husbands do on a daily basis, like leaving dirty washing everywhere but in the washing machine, empty boxes without any food left in them still in the pantry or fridge, not replacing the empty toilet roll, and the list could go on and on. I use to share funny stuff that Ray did that drove me insane, and not that I knew it at the time, but it made me concentrate on how bloody annoying that little thing was because I was putting more energy into it than necessary. I would harp on about it to friends and we'd have our little bitch about how hopeless our husbands can be, but again we were just feeding the negativity, so it would multiply faster than the coronavirus. Once I started to shift my energy to more positive thoughts and focus on what I was grateful for in my life, the negative thoughts seemed to disappear and stop overcrowding my mind. I became more receptive of others' negativity too, and instead of feeding it, alarm bells would ring and I would change the subject or remove myself from the conversation. Of course I still have negative thoughts, I'm no Mother Teresa by any means, but if I don't feed them by saying them out loud and giving them the time of day, they tend to get bored and just pack their bags for a new home.

With negative thoughts also comes judgement. I was so hard on myself and others that my judgement ruled my mind. I remember visiting my nan when we were kids, and her house was always immaculate. She would be down on hands and knees mopping the bathroom floor every morning after everyone had finished showering. You'd never see a dirty pile of clothes on her laundry floor or would you ever find a pile of clean clothes needing to be folded up and put away on the couch or kitchen table. Growing up I believed a clean and spotless house was the representation of a good, happy home. It made me judge anyone's home that was far from perfect, and that included my own. I had unrealistic expectations of myself and of the rest of the world.

Before I had kids, I was on one of those women whose *house wouldn't look like that, my kids would never do that, as a mother I wouldn't do that*, but it is so easy to judge from the outside of a world you've never experienced yourself. Putting ridiculous expectations on myself to have the perfect home took its toll on me, and I was living to get every little chore done before I could enjoy life. Household chores, as we know, are endless, leaving me no time to enjoy the perfect home I had created, and to add to that I'd obsess about anyone messing it up. It wasn't pleasant for me or my family. Now, I'm not saying for us all to live like complete pigs, but no-one's going to care about the state of your house when they visit if they are a true friend. If they do, it's more of a reflection of them than you. And if you find yourself judging someone else, ask yourself why. And are those thoughts more of an insight into yourself rather than the person you are focusing your negative energy on?

CONTROL FREAK

We've all heard the old saying, 'Well, we can see who wears the pants in your relationship.' Ray and I still get it at work now, even though it is far from the truth. There are things that each of us do better—organisation isn't Ray's strength but I live for it, hence why I organise all our finances. In no way is it so that I can control what he spends—he can buy whatever he likes as long as we can afford it at the time—but things just didn't get paid when they were under his responsibility.

I used to be a controlling partner; I'd probably go as far as to say I was overbearing. I hated when Ray went out with the boys or left me at any time. I was scared I wouldn't cope being home with both the boys with no adult interaction. And how come he got to go have all the fun whilst I was stuck at home with the kids? His life hadn't been affected at all since having children—that's the way I thought back then, because my mind was so unhealthy. I had FOMO, big time! I had to be in control of everything and everyone. I think this is why motherhood was such a challenge for me, because as we all know, children are unpredictable and uncontrollable. When Ray wasn't home, I had no control of what he was up to, and he was shit at keeping in contact when he wasn't home, which made the situation even worse. What I couldn't see at the time is how bloody lucky I was to have a husband who didn't want to get shitfaced every weekend at the pub with his mates and blow a shitload of money; his idea of fun is a shooting or fishing trip, sleeping in his swag around a campfire with his mates, and a few too many beers. Ray had become reluctant to ask me if he could go on trips like these because of my constant negative reaction, and instead stopped planning them. It's now that I can see it's trips like these that he needed for his own mental health, and I was depriving him of them for so long for my own selfishness and inability to let go due to my poor mental state. These days I enjoy the times when he is away on his boys' trips; I know that I am more than capable of looking after the boys on my own, and to be honest, they are better behaved when it's just the three of us. We also have a much happier dad and husband, which is all we could dream for.

SELF-LOVE

Thirty-six years it has taken me to love myself, cellulite and all! For thirty-six years I've expected and wanted people to love someone who not even I could love. I was toxic on the inside and, like a volcano erupting, my toxic insides would ooze out like lava from my mouth when I spoke, and in my mind when I thought. I would look in the mirror and only see something that wasn't good enough, far from perfection, far from the face and body I had had years before, no longer young and taut. How is it that I could find beauty in an image of a confident curvy woman but not see the same when my appearance was similar? Anything bigger than a size ten and I was fat in my eyes. I would dissect every single photo that I was in and delete the majority of them if I looked in any way what I thought was fat or ugly—this even included photos with my boys. My own insecurities flowed into my relationships and made me think I would always be cheated on, because I was never good enough, never perfect, never just enough for someone.

I have battled with my relationship with food all my life. I am the queen of fad diets, yo-yo dieting and binge eating. I have the will power to stick to something short-term and get the instant results, but it was never a lifestyle I could maintain. And to be honest, I love delicious food. But on the other hand, I use food to punish myself in a way. I don't know why this is, but I can get in the mindset of just having to eat until I am physically ill for no goddamn reason. Then I get all down and out afterwards and the cycle goes on. Since the easing of restrictions from the pandemic, I signed up to a local privately owned gym. My personal trainer, who is also the owner, has educated me about nutrition and made me understand it more clearly, especially the tricks behind the fad diets that never last. She doesn't write out a generalised food plan for her members because she knows one plan that works for one person won't necessarily work for the next. She works one on one with her clients to build something that works for them, suits their lifestyle, and, most importantly, is something they can stick to long-term. Her no-bullshit approach has me scared to never no-show to a class or cancel last minute. This is the longest I have been committed to my health and wellbeing for a long time, and I'm feeling the positive benefits.

Before I could concentrate on me, though, I had to get the rest of my life sorted. If you are surrounded by chaos, you are likely to feel chaotic. It took moving interstate to get a work-life balance, moving again closer to work and a town for easy access to a gym and less travel time to and from work, plus making sure Ray and the boys were happy, before I could put one hundred percent commitment into myself and finally stick to it. Hallelujah!

TRIGGERS

Anyone and everyone can suffer from a form of mental illness; how severe and debilitating it can be on that person may depend. Being able to work out what triggers my anxiety and what helps reduce it has helped a lot over the years since I've been on medication.

Speaking to a psychiatrist once, she told me anxiety causes you to have an unrealistic expectation of the world, a need for everything to be perfect. And, of course, we all know nothing is ever perfect, especially us as humans. But knowing that doesn't stop my mind from expecting it, particularly of myself.

One of the things that I know I can do to help reduce my anxiety is putting self-care at the top of my to-do list. Looking after myself physically improves my outlook on the world. Eating a healthy diet and exercising regularly makes my outlook on the world more positive. 'Strong body, strong mind' is my favourite positive affirmation. Even though it's not the case for everyone, it is for me at this moment. I know that if I can stay committed to strengthening my body externally, strength will flow internally through to my mind as well.

As women, our bodies go through different hormonal changes throughout the period of a month. Some forms of contraception will also mess with our body's natural level of certain hormones. I found it impossible to find a contraceptive pill that worked for me during the time between the two boys being born, even though I had been on the same pill since my late teens before I had Brayden. We all know the dreaded PMS we get the week before our periods; well, some pills would make that week unbearable for me. I'd completely lose my shit and feel like I couldn't go on. My anxiety went through the roof and I was impossible to live with. Another pill made me feel like that all month round, and in the end I just couldn't deal with the ups and downs. I am no longer on any form of contraceptive, but my body still experiences all the natural hormonal changes that women go through, and I know where my cycle is at every month due to how I am feeling mentally. My anxiety can flare up at certain times of the month, but being more aware of the stages my body is at in terms of my menstrual cycle has helped wonders. It is clearly obvious when I'm a week out from my period, because my OCD goes through the roof: every little annoying thing that my husband does becomes a thousand times more annoying, and the sound of chewing actually sends me off the rails, especially when it is coming from him. Men should understand that women don't even want them to breathe near them during the PMS stage. I also crave time on my own, without the noise of the kids or the constant questions from my husband, even if it's just Ray putting the boys to bed so I can sit and watch some TV on my own. I have the need to just hide away from the world during these days and allow my body to just do its thing.

Distraction is a killer for my anxiety. This is where I find social media comes into play. I'll find myself mindlessly reloading social media apps to keep my focus on anything else but the present. Some distraction in life is necessary, like cooking dinner and other household chores that your kids just won't let you do without nagging at your feet, driving you absolutely bonkers! But I find I can now filter out and be more aware of the unnecessary distractions like social media, and put them aside to concentrate on the kids or the job at hand to reduce my levels of anxiety.

Alcohol! I love being the life of the party, and even though I've never felt like I've been on the verge of classing myself as an alcoholic, I don't think my relationship with alcohol has always been a healthy one. I'm a serial binge drinker, to the point where I won't remember everything from the night before. This, straight away, isn't good for my anxiety, as I worry if I did something stupid, if I embarrassed myself, if I said the wrong thing to the wrong person. So, I sit and stew for days after digging myself back into a dark hole. When I drink, I also eat way too much of all the wrong foods that seem like a great idea at the time. I'll get up the following day, feel sorry for myself all day, eat more crappy food and definitely won't even consider doing any form of exercise, and the bad cycle will continue from there. Since being on a lifestyle roster, where we get four to five days off at a time, I've noticed I'll drink heavily for more days in a row, so any routine I had goes out the window. It's only been the last six weeks, at the end of isolation, that I've finally got my shit into gear. I love exercising again, rather than feeling like it is a chore. I've lost the excess weight that's stopped me from fitting into my clothes, and I've cut down my drinking to one or two here and there, but mainly on a special occasion. I was even the designated driver recently for a friend's birthday party, and I felt bloody amazing the next day. Progress, not perfection!

Communication is the Achilles heel to my marriage to Ray, and probably is to a lot of relationships. I have the tendency to bottle everything up, as I get sick of wasting my time talking to a brick wall. Over time, all the little annoying things Ray does or doesn't do build up, and my anxiety replays them a hundred times over and over in my head. It plays out conversations I wish I could just have with him, to scream at him, to the point where I just want to explode, and normally I do get to that point, and that's when Ray finally sees that he's pushed me over the edge and starts making an effort. It always feels a little bit too late by then.

Let's just say that my husband, in general, as much as I love him, is a major trigger for my anxiety. I hate that when I'm frustrated at him the boys are the ones who cop my impatience, because I'm already at a heightened level of anxiety and I just can't deal with any more shit.

The boys stir my anxiety continually, but never on purpose. They make the simplest things seem so difficult, like eating their dinner, or listening the first time they're told no so I don't have to go all Hulk-Mum on them (as they call it). In my head, I repeatedly say, *How fucking hard is it, kids? We do this shit every* day*; it's part of everyday life; why does it need to be so hard?* Brayden has this thing where he holds on to go to the toilet to the very last second. He can hold on to number one and two like it's an Olympic sport. I know he needs to go because he dances around like there's ants in his pants, or keeps squeezing his doodle until I'm afraid it might drop off, but the more I ask him, the more he denies it. It frustrates the fuck out of me! Seriously, mate, it can't be comfortable holding on that long. Kids can make the simplest thing seem like such a drama, and at times it can be difficult to handle.

WILL I EVER BE HIS PRIORITY?

Throughout this book, I have touched on times when I haven't felt like Ray has been there for me like a husband ideally would be, and I've never felt like I have ever been top of his priority list. Over the space of our relationship, I have felt continually let down by Ray. Sometimes it has been over big things, other times it's just little things on a day-to-day basis. But when they all build up over the years, I have grown to form a fear and an acceptance that Ray will always let me down.

We are at a stage where we are looking at attending couples counselling again. Not because we are at breaking point, but because we need to work through things, like those I have mentioned above, so that small issues don't turn into long-term resentment, because once resentment sets in it's bloody hard to come back from.

For some people, counselling is a last resort; for us, it's preventing it from getting to that stage. Communication is the weakest link in our marriage, and we are going around in circles, having the same conversation with no results. Sometimes it's good to have that mediator there so you can have the courage to say things you find hard to say to each other's faces, worried of the reaction.

We still love each other and find each other sexually attractive, which is a huge bonus, because that is something that can dwindle over the years, once children are introduced and you both change both physically and emotionally. My grandparents have always taught us kids that a healthy sex life is the key to a successful marriage, and they are living proof that it helps.

I read a quote the other day: 'Don't just settle for someone who loves you. Find someone who's capable of being the teammate you need in life', and this resonated deep down for me. We talk about our husbands being the biggest child of the house, and it can be funny at times, but it's not what is going to grow a long and prosperous marriage. It's exhausting, and no woman wants to take the place of their husband's mum in their life—do we, ladies. And, in time, it's going to build resentment, and that's where I am at the moment.

Ray is, and always will be, the man of my dreams. I still look at him and find him as sexy as ever and wonder how I got so lucky. I'll do everything and anything to strengthen our marriage and build it to be what we both want and need in life, taking it one day at a time.

TAKING THE GOOD WITH THE BAD

If I'm completely honest, mental illness is something I believe I'm going to have to manage for the rest of my life. I don't think it will just magically go away one day. Even though my long-term goal is to manage it without the assistance of medication, I'm in no way ready to go it alone without any medical support anytime soon.

As with every human being, I still have my up and down days, but thankfully the downer days are becoming fewer and further in between.

With the assistance of meditation, I am becoming more conscious of those down times and can accept them for what they are and allow my body to ride through the motions before coming out on the other side, back to my normal cheery self again. Some days I just want to sleep and hide away from the world. I screen calls and messages, even from my closest friends and family, because I can't get my head around stringing a conversation together. Ray can sense the times I am more withdrawn—it's generally when my hormones are all over the shop—and he knows I just need to let it pass and it is in no way a reflection of how we are at the time or anything he has done.

Work seems to be somewhere I can strive daily. No matter how much shit I am dealing with, I can fake it until I make it at work. I don't know why that is. I recently changed from operating dump trucks to co-ordinating the pit. With it has come longer hours and more stress and responsibility, but somehow it's an environment I've thrived in. Maybe this is because my mind is so used to functioning in fight-or-flight mode, or perhaps it's because I'd live or die for organisation. Since taking the position I feel like it's given me more work satisfaction too, and a sense of accomplishment each day, which is something I crave from any career path I choose. My position requires me to fly by the seat of my pants and is forever changing and unpredictable, a little bit like motherhood, so I feel like it's helping me learn how to cope and manage situations at home better as well. The downside to being in fight-or-flight mode frequently is the high levels of cortisone being pumped through my body, which we all know more commonly as the stress hormone. High levels of cortisone means I hold on to fluid more then I'd like and I stress-eat sugary, crappy foods to keep up with the rush. Afterwards I feel shit and bloated and, just like the effects of a mind-altering drug, what goes up must come down, and I find I spend the first day or two off work recovering from the week and feeling absolutely exhausted and withdrawn sometimes, just needing to rest and reset.

MY VILLAGERS

In this book, I have mentioned people who have helped to make up my village, and the importance of having a village around you for support when you have children.

To the mum-to-be whom I first met in antenatal classes, my newborn photographer who became a dear friend, all the girls from my mothers' group, my workmates, my Melbourne GFs, my family, Ray's family and anyone else who has crossed our paths over the last five years, thank you from the bottom of my heart for offering support and unconditional love to our little family.

I haven't yet mentioned three very important villagers in this book who have been helpful to us by being there for the boys and me in good times and bad: my bestie Moo Moo (long story on the nickname) and my brother and sister-in-law.

My brother and sister-in-law welcomed me into their family with open arms from the first time I met them. Their marriage is one I looked up to, and their realistic approach to parenting still reassures me that I'm doing OK. My sister-in-law said to me during the time I was struggling with my mental health, 'You've got to look after you, no-one else is,' and she was so bloody right. No one was looking out for me, so it was up to me to get some help and turn my life around. Thank you both for everything.

Lucky last is my bestie, Moo Moo. We have known each other since we met working in Heaven Nightclub in Adelaide in our early twenties. Our friendship has had its ups and downs, and there have been times when we haven't been as close as we are today since both starting families. In the sixteen years we have been friends, we have lived in the same city for only a few of them. We are polar opposites when it comes to being mums, but coincidently we both had two boys. She dresses her boys only in monochrome colours and, more then often, with matching outfits, whereas my kids wear all the colours of the rainbow, and my type of matchy-matchy is the boys sporting the same superhero jumper. We have an ongoing joke where I send her photos of the boys' outfits and she expresses how much all that colour hurts her eyes. It's everything a friendship should be. She is my rock. We speak daily, if not five times a day, and say 'I love you' when we say goodbye. We don't judge each other; we lay shit on each other and we support each other no matter what happens in our lives. We motivate each other, and strive to be the best we can with everything in our lives because we know we can. We cry and we laugh together. I couldn't imagine my village without her. Since moving to NSW, and with our boys being a little bit older, we have been able to catch up for little mum getaways and they are the highlight of my year. We may not be related by blood, but she is my sister through and through. Friendships like these are hard to find, and I know I'll treasure this one until the day I die.

THE END

Writing this book has been a form of therapy for me, to be able to accept, heal and leave the past in the past where it belongs. Putting everything down onto paper and reliving it all has made me realise that *wow*, it has been a hectic past five or so years. However, I've come out the other end stronger than I've ever been or felt before, and have handled everything life has thrown at me (but only just!).

I shared my book with a handful of my dearest friends once I had completed it. Most of the feedback was positive, an appreciation of my honesty to share things they themselves have experienced but never spoken about. One very honest friend came back with the feedback that the book sounded resentful towards my husband, and I had the choice to accept and love him for who he is or leave him. I was shocked at first, but then I remembered that the truth can sometimes hurt. I drank a lot that night and cried more than I had in a long time, thinking about what this all meant. I came to the realisation that she and I have a very different perspective when it comes to relationships and how to balance them. And even though I appreciate her honesty, I feel Ray and I still have a long way to come for a long and happy marriage, but we are not at the beginning of the end; there are things we can work on as a team without losing ourselves or breaking up. It's about compromising and deciding on some non-negotiables we have for each other. It's about disconnecting from our phones and reconnecting with each other. It's about daily communication. I know love is not everything when it comes to a lasting relationship, but it's a bloody good starting point, and there's no-one else I would want to do life with but Ray. I've reread the book over and over after receiving that feedback, trying to reword anything I felt painted my husband in a bad light. In no way is this book an attack on him; this book is written for him. It's my cry for help to him. It's everything we haven't been able to talk about. It's experiencing the past five years through my eyes, and I appreciate that he is taking the time to read it, for it's a step in the right direction: forward.

I am still of two minds on how the general public will receive this book. The ones that I have confided in throughout the writing process to give me honest feedback have loved it. Maybe that's because they know me personally. The world is a nasty place these days, especially online, so I worry that the judgement and trolling will be unbearable to cope with, because this is seriously my life out there for the whole world to read, warts and all. But deep down I want to be brave enough to kill the stigma towards mental health and make those who have or haven't experienced the torture of it know that it could affect them or anyone they know, or, even worse, someone they are very close to could be living through it right now without them having any awareness of it. I want to give the women and men out there the courage to seek help, to know it's OK if you are finding motherhood, marriage, or even life in general too hard, because things are not always a walk in the park, especially not life at times, but I hope that we can all get through it with some support and love around us.

There are so many free support lines out there for everyone and anyone to reach out for help. If you know someone who is struggling, reach out to them again and again, even if they push you away. Be persistent. You could be the light at the end of the tunnel that saves their life one day.

EPILOGUE

I don't think anyone's 2020 New Year's resolution would've included surviving a worldwide coronavirus pandemic, the possibility of being unemployed, or enduring extended times of isolation with our kids and husbands. I'm not one to make New Year's resolutions, as they generally end up being the things I don't stick to that year, and, let's be honest, majority are clique like 'lose weight', 'quit smoking', etc, things we could focus our energy on anytime of the year but instead decide the busiest time of the year when we all drink, eat and party too much is a great time to start. Plus most of us still have a month of school holidays to survive, so let's be kind to ourselves and set goals that may be more achievable. Alcohol-free school holidays are really a stretch for any mother.

In all seriousness, whilst I was able to utilise the isolation period to write about my experiences with living with mental illness, the world is experiencing an unprecedented rise in poor mental health due to the current economic circumstances. Now more than ever is this the time to reach out and ask, 'Are you OK?'

My main goal for this book was that my husband Ray would read it and we would live happily ever after, like in the movies. Before this book, the longest thing my husband had read would have been an article in a fishing magazine, but slowly he chipped away at my book. I am forever grateful, and it meant the absolute world to me that he took time to do something that was so out of his comfort zone, but that he knew meant so much to me. After, he complimented me on the achievement whilst being very much surprised that I could string a word or two together. Most importantly, he gave me permission to share our story, if that was what I wanted to do. This was so brave of him, as a man, and to be OK with sharing his own battles with mental health with the world speaks volumes.

Ray and I still haven't gone back to couples counselling; we solely worked on ourselves first, and when we were ready, we escaped for a weekend away, smashed down the wall of emotions between us (plus a few too many bottles of wine) and just talked. We spoke about things from the past, present and future. We chatted about everything and anything. We took turns to really listen to each other, and it was the most proactive conversation we have ever had. Maybe we were both in a position to finally hear each other out without judgement. Our list of non-negotiables and the promise that weekend to openly communicate with each other daily has stuck in place ever since, and our relationship and house is a much happier place at the moment.

The 'big O' is a more frequent occurrence in my life now when Ray and I make love. The changes I have been continually working on to improve myself both physically and mentally have definitely paid off in the bedroom. Constant changes in our routines from working a rotating roster with long hours means we may not sleep together daily, but when we do it's passionate and intimate.

My non-existence on social media had me wondering how I could possibly market a book or connect with readers so once again I have caved into the addiction that is social media and my alcohol intake is back to being up and down like a yoyo. My current life moto is progress not perfection as I battle with bad habits I have dealt with for most of my life.

After months of research and contemplating, I finally decided to invest in myself and took the leap of faith to self-publish my book. The joys of self-publishing meant I had full control over all the creative decisions of the book, and even though graphic design for the cover was included, I wanted it to be more personal than that. My best friend had suggested the art of continuous line drawings to capture the emotions of the book in illustration. I stumbled across the amazing work created by Samantha Lentini. She had created a custom piece for someone I admire, and I just knew as soon as I scrolled through her posts that she was the perfect artist to portray my story. After contacting Sam, I knew I had made the right decision. She was lovely and encouraging, and she just got my concept straight away. Thank you, Sam, for putting my words into pictures.

And thank you in advance to anyone who takes the time to read my story. I hope you find it as interesting as it was for me to live.

CPSIA information can be obtained
at www.ICGtesting.com
Printed in the USA
LVHW081543230323
742311LV00025B/1419

9 780228 844891